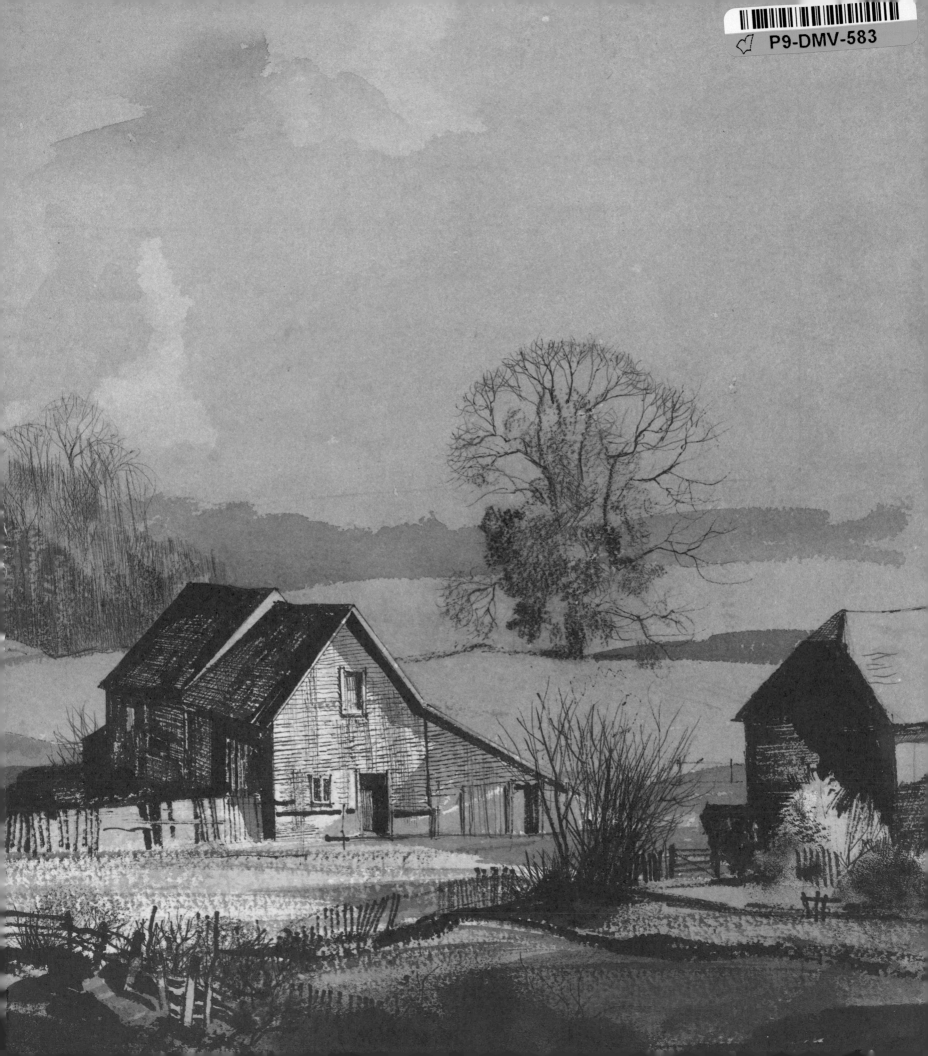

ROWLAND HILDER COUNTRY

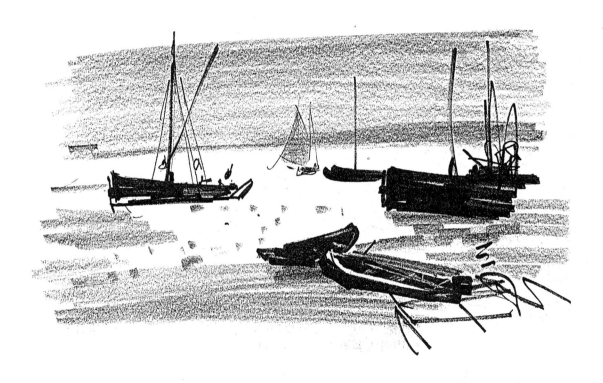

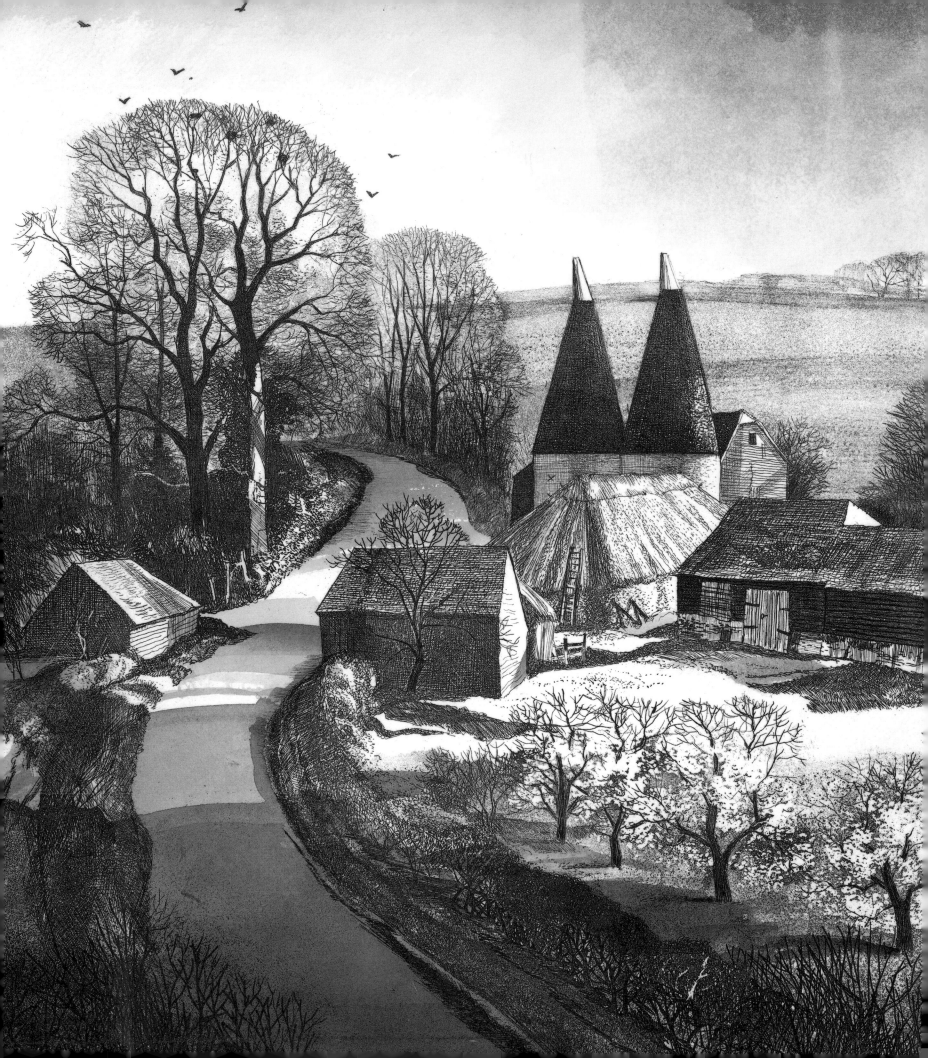

ROWLAND HILDER COUNTRY

An artist's memoir
edited by Denis Thomas

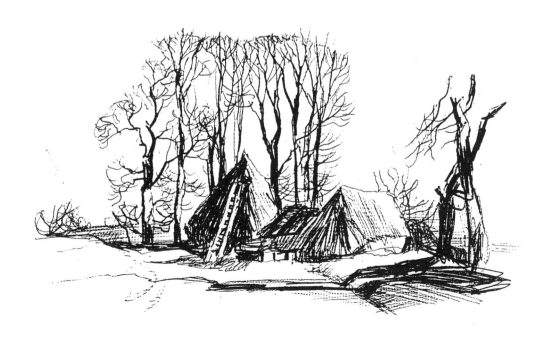

THE HERBERT PRESS

Copyright © Rowland Hilder and Denis Thomas 1987
Copyright under the Berne Convention

First published in Great Britain 1987 by
The Herbert Press Ltd, 46 Northchurch Road, London N1 4EJ
Reprinted 1988

Designed by Pauline Harrison
Colour photography by Rado Klose
Colour separations by Royle Print
Typeset by Butler & Tanner Ltd, Frome
Printed and bound in Hong Kong by South China Printing Co.

British Library Cataloguing in Publication Data:
Hilder, Rowland
    Rowland Hilder country: an artist's memoir.
    1. Hilder, Rowland
    I. Title   II. Thomas, Denis
    759.2   ND497.H57/
ISBN 0–906969–74–3

FRONTISPIECE
A detail from *The Garden of England*, re-worked as an etching, 1987.

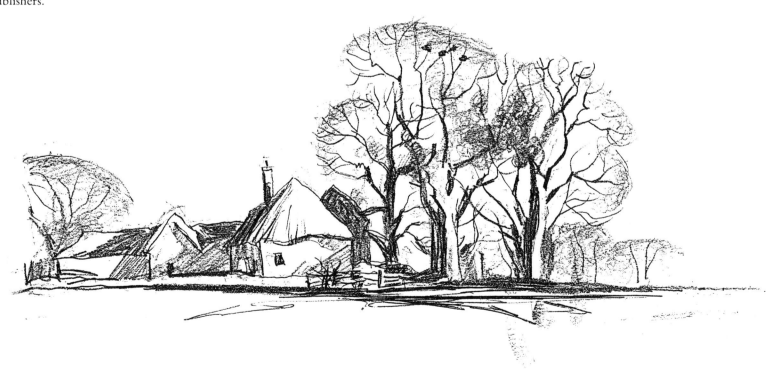

Contents

Foreword 6

Time and Place 17

Town and Around 37

Banks and Braes 63

Four Seasons 79

Quiet Waters 99

Pen and Pencil 113

Bibliography 127

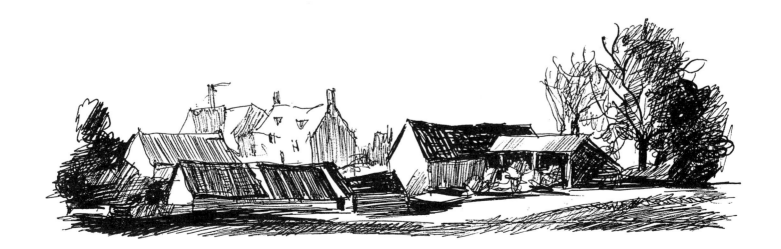

Foreword

The reception given to *Rowland Hilder's England* has been, for me, one of the heart-warming experiences of my life. Any communicator likes to feel that he is in touch with that great unknown quantity, the British public. To do so through the medium of painting is an exceptional privilege. This second 'retrospective' enlarges on the events, ideas and circumstances that have helped to keep me busy, as an artist, into my eighties, and also introduces some examples of my latest work. Once again I am pleased to acknowledge the contribution of Royles, the printers and publishers, with whom I have enjoyed a long and productive association. To all friends, whether known to us or not, Edith and I extend the hope that they will share our pleasure in making this book.

ROWLAND HILDER

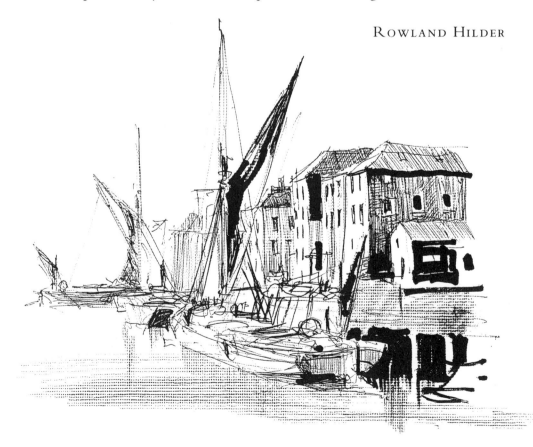

6

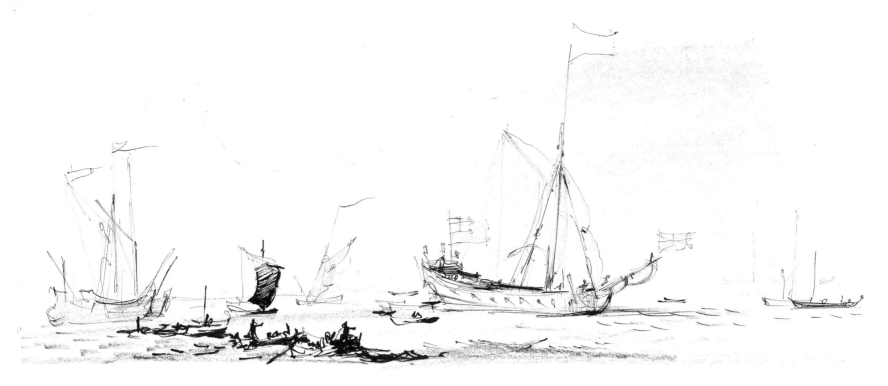

I did not know it at the time, but one of the first people I ever held a serious conversation with was a millionaire picture-collector, Andrew Mellon, the American tycoon whose son was to become such an enthusiast for English art that he formed the world's best private collection of it, from Stubbs and Gainsborough to Cox and De Wint. Mr Mellon Snr was one of my father's contacts in New York, where he, my mother and I were living in an apartment off Central Park. I cannot be sure if Mr Mellon and I discussed the fine arts (I was about six years old at the time), but according to my mother our little chats made an impression on him. 'I like talking to that young chap,' he told her. 'I get more sense out of him than I do out of most grown-ups.'

We were a thoroughly English little family, despite the circumstance of my being born at Great Neck, Long Island, in 1905. My name was misspelt on the registration form (it was not meant to have a 'w' in it), but that version stuck and we soon got used to it. I went to school in Morristown, New Jersey, when my parents left New York, and acquired a good American accent that tended to mark me out on our trips back to England every summer. I eventually came back for good aboard the *Lusitania* in 1915, the last voyage she made before the U-boats sent her to the bottom. My father, from our safe base in the United States, had decided that the Old Country needed him, and he was not a man to let the enemy-infested ocean come between him and his patriotic duty. I remember the crossing vividly, as I do all the earlier ones. Sailing the Atlantic in those days was an exciting experience for any youngster, and I have an idea that my lifelong feeling for ships and the sea dates from those voyages across the mighty waterway.

I was parked with my grandparents at Birling, in Kent, not far from Maidstone. To me it seemed miles from anywhere. Even the people living in the next village to us, Ryarsh, were considered as foreigners. My grandparents, of course, had no car, and my first glimpse of the Kent countryside, so familiar to generations of Hilders from those parts, was from a horse and buggy. I was used to horses, and to travelling around in this fashion, because in America we had had the run of Mr Mellon's rolling acres. In the Kentish countryside, crisscrossed with lanes, there were relatives to visit on every side, and these first impressions of our native county were not lost on me. My father, a dedicated amateur painter, then bought a splendid old car with oil lamps and a klaxon horn and a thing called a dickey seat, where I was strapped in, wearing goggles against the weather. He used to take me with him on his sketching excursions along the narrow lanes, pulling up at likely spots. If you looked back you could see the way we had come: clouds of dust hung between the hedgerows, marking our winding way.

My father liked to look at pictures wherever we went. He was knowledgeable about the Impressionists, whose works he had seen in the homes of Mr Mellon and his circle. That was unusual for the time, since there were as yet practically none to be seen in England: he was fortunate to have had access to them in the only city, apart from Paris, where there were any to be seen. I remember him showing me some Whistler etchings in one of these habitations, the American equivalent of a stately home. My first sniff of oil paint was in a room where one of these notables, a banker or railway magnate perhaps, was having his portrait painted.

After the war, from which my father returned safe and sound, we went to live at a tobacconist's shop in New Cross which he had bought on enlisting in the Royal Horse Artillery, for my mother to run if the Germans got him. I was sent to a local boys' school, where I did not exactly shine as a scholar, and spent as much time as I could simply drawing. The art master, looking at my sketches, told my parents that the best place for me was an art college. While I was waiting for that happy day, I began to explore the nearby Thames between the Surrey docks and the Royal Naval College at Greenwich. It was alive with activity; smelly, noisy, oily, with men's shouts sounding above the cry of the gulls. It captivated me. I could not stop drawing it all: tugs, colliers, shipboard tackle, amazing rigging, taut, snapping sails, hooters, sirens, men rolling barrels, the tang of tar and the creeping promise of the sea. I longed for the skill to put it all down.

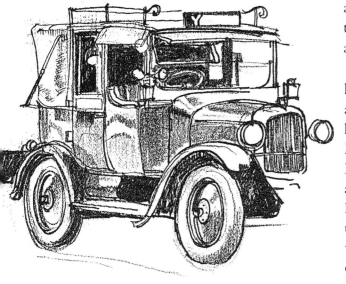

Then, at last, I was admitted to Goldsmiths'. I would set out from our little home at the tobacconist's shop every morning, on foot or by tram. I was sixteen, and though my teachers had marked me out as a possible draughtsman I still had everything to learn. They put me in the etching class, which was run by Malcolm Osborne, an ARA who had been a pupil of the great Frank Short. Etching at that time was regarded as an accomplishment that could provide an artist with a livelihood, for there were still enough collectors to make a market. However, after making a start I abandoned etching for illustration. It turned out to be a good decision, if only because the etching boom, had we but known it, was on the wane, obliging several outstanding young artists to look for other careers. I had acquired, however, a knowledge of the medium which has lain dormant until recent times, when it has provided me with an additional means of expression by enabling me to re-work some of my most characteristic subjects as etchings, ranging from softgrounds to aquatints, and recently introducing the heretical element of colour. In developing these traditional crafts in modern terms I have had at my side the talents, and necessary muscle, of my son-in-law, Rado Klose: an exercise in family teamwork which we both enjoy.

In the illustration class at Goldsmiths' I found an inspiring teacher in Edmund J. Sullivan, one of the generation of black-and-white artists that included the likes of Phil May, Tom Browne and Aubrey Beardsley. He led us away from classroom life-drawing towards rapid action sketches, using the sketch-pad as a reporter uses his notebook, always at hand, whatever the subject. Academic accuracy could wait: the essential thing, Sullivan kept telling us, was to catch the passing scene. One thing one learns as time passes is that dogmas and the received wisdom of teachers and art scholars are ephemeral. But Sullivan's ideas, and his example, are with me still.

The first English artists I studied were marine painters such as W. L. Wyllie and Charles Dixon. Brangwyn, at the time, had his adherents also, and one of my fellow students, Graham Sutherland, persuaded me to look at him more closely. I did so; and he became a bridge by which I was able to make the crossing from one skill, drawing, to another that I already aspired to, painting. Meanwhile, I was awarded a travelling scholarship, which offered a chance to sharpen my eye on unfamiliar places. Instead of going to Italy to gaze on the old masters, however, I reckoned I would derive more benefit from sailing in a tramp steamer across the North Sea, then up the canals into the heart of Europe. Earlier this year I came across one of the drawings I brought home from that trip, a watercolour of Flushing. It must have been one of my first, and I looked at it with some interest. Whatever its merits, it reminded me how, at that stage in my life, it had been virtually impossible to learn how to use watercolour. Sixty years ago it was not on any art school's curriculum: it had been swept aside by the arrival from Europe of the Modern Movement, whose aims did not lend themselves to our gentle, subtle, understated English medium. Everything that I felt tended in the opposite direction from these imported 'isms'. I was for observation, naturalism, and the traditions of the English School.

I was a trained draughtsman; but ambition went further than that. Perhaps I could get into marine painting, given my abiding love of sea subjects? But no – marine artists in the Twenties and Thirties were romantics, strong on sailing ships battling round the Horn or sitting serenely in a tropical sunset. I did try selling my marine drawings of boats in dock or fitting-out in the Port of London. But the dealers kept telling me that they only wanted work like the popular Arthur Briscoe's, of the 'heeling clipper' kind. That was the market, and I was not in it.

Meanwhile, despairing of finding anyone to teach me how to paint in water-colour, I had no alternative but to try and teach myself. Doing it oneself proved to be a painfully slow grind, with terrible results. I was getting nowhere: any

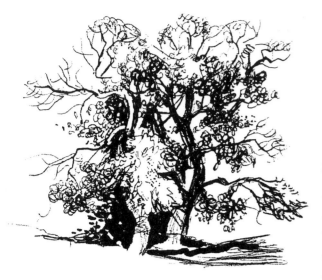

amateur today, in a totally different art climate, would make a better job of it than I did. It was a long time before I came anywhere near mastering the art, and I do not like to dwell on the efforts of those early days. However, well into middle age I was admitted to the Royal Institute of Painters in Water Colours, and in due course they made me President.

My life had taken a decisive turn, meanwhile, when Jonathan Cape commissioned me to illustrate a special edition of *Precious Bane*, that enormously popular novel by Mary Webb, in 1928. The story has been told many times, but at the risk of repeating a familiar legend let me just say that the experience of working as an artist in the depths of an English winter opened my eyes to an aspect of landscape painting which, so far as I could see, no English painter had tackled before. It was an opportunity to look at landscape that appealed to my draughtsman's eye – showing the bare bones of winter – and to set off, at last, on the road to becoming a painter.

If it is any encouragement to a reader of these words, the lesson is that if you would like to paint, give yourself half a lifetime to make it. When Edith and I first went to the States together and showed some pictures, one woman wanted to know how long it took me to do one of my paintings. (Americans, you understand, need to know how much everybody earns or makes: it gives them an idea of one's standing in relation to the dollar.) We could not answer this. So in the end we worked out that a single picture might take nine months from conception to delivery, the same gestation time as for our questioner. This answer seemed acceptable; it did not even raise a smile.

But creating a painting can be a long-drawn-out process. Between the idea and the finished work there lies a succession of stages, not all of them under complete control, since there is usually a point at which the painting becomes obstinate and insists on going its own way. The artist may be obliged to have half a dozen stabs at it before it is ready to let him go. One advantage of this protracted process is that a subject that has put the painter through the mill tends to give him the most satisfaction when it is over. This applies even when the subject is one he has tackled before. Every repetition is, in fact, another variant on an inexhaustible theme.

One of the difficulties, or realities, of having worked right through the twentieth century so far (I am not threatening to go on working through the next!) is that in that span of time I have had to confine painting to the intervals between making a more conventional living, in the commercial world – where all of us end up unless we are born with lots of money – and as a teacher. Also, while working within a tradition, I have been very conscious of the pressure of modern schools, changing media, technical advances in materials, and market changes which help to keep the art world on its toes. Looking outside the academic world, I found a few artists whose work was based on draughtsmanship but who also mastered my favoured medium, watercolour, among them Muirhead Bone and Henry Rushbury. But we were an isolated few.

If people regard my landscapes as in some way 'nostalgic' it is because so many of them originated a generation or two ago, before mechanisation took over from husbandry and before suburbia overwhelmed the vision of green fields at the bottom of everybody's garden; before diesel engines knocked out sail, and containers knocked out the docks.

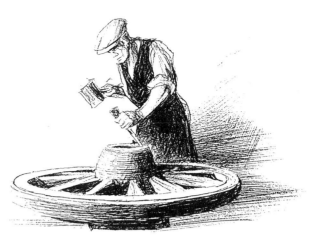

There is something one learns from people's reactions to one's work as it gradually becomes better known. It is that the satisfaction they express, often very pleasing for a painter to hear, is not so much in the picture they have in mind as in their own recollection – what the picture reminds them of. The scene they are so strongly drawn to may very well not exist – it has been re-worked in the creative process of making it into a picture. What people say they like about a particular painting, because it stirs some memory or distant feeling, may not be credited to the painter every time: the response is already waiting there, for the artist's touch. So many people have told me that certain places I have painted were where they once lived, or near where they got married, or where their parents used to take them when they were children. They ask me to locate the place for them, help them to get back to it. Over and again I have to disappoint them. The picture is 'true', but there is no such place. It has passed through someone else's mind, imagination, call it what you like, to where it now sits, on a piece of paper. An evocative painting may be just an agency by which other people's feelings are brought to the surface. There is another factor at work here, too: the extent to which a painting in progress can at some stage begin to go its own way, as I described earlier. With watercolour, of course, once that happens the painter has to let it, because with watercolour you don't get a second chance. But I would put all that conjecture aside for the sake of the feeling one gets when one's tussle with the medium comes out right.

The general conception of painting a watercolour is that you take your paints and brushes and drawing board out into the countryside, look round for a subject, then sit down and start it. Things are not that simple. Rather than sitting down and painting literally what my eyes tell me is there in front of me, I search for the essence of the time and place. I cannot begin until that starting point is clear to me. Mere places do not make pictures; except for the photographer, unless one's response to them is something more than automatic.

Like everyone else, I have been attracted by places which are known to be 'picturesque' and where a well-known paintable scene is waiting. Willy Lott's Cottage is an example – the best-known corner of the Constable country by the Suffolk Stour, which you can see in the great *Hay Wain* and many other paintings by him which are part of our mental store of picturesque subjects. The difficulty is that such places already bear such a load of associations that it is only rarely that one is able to experience a personal response rather than a second-hand one. On the other hand, subjects which by most standards offer little of the picturesque, such as the inside of a barn or a street corner in some busy township, can and do provoke the artist into getting out his sketchbook and pencil. What one draws is so often just a matter of where one happens to be. When I am visiting people, the drawings I bring back are likely to be interiors. When I am on the edge of the sea they are likely to be random scenes of messing about in boats, with all the clobber and untidiness familiar to boating people, rather like domestic scenes at home, in working areas such as the kitchen or the scruffy end of the garden. These are individual rather than well-worn responses to places we feel at home in, liking them as they are, not prettied-up to make a conventionally engaging picture.

The Shoreham Valley, which is at the heart of what people now call the Samuel Palmer country, is also at the heart of much of my work. When I was a student it was the nearest accessible stretch of countryside. You could go down by train, alighting at the little station behind the church, or, as I did, by bicycle. The Goldsmiths' students knew it well, long before Samuel Palmer came into our ken. The sudden awareness that this was the hallowed ground of a visionary English artist certainly made it more interesting, but that came later. None of us, as youngsters, had even heard of him. One artist who did know his work, and was deep in research into it, was F. L. Griggs, the masterly illustrator of many of the classic 'Highways and Byways' series covering the English counties, published in the first decade of the century by Macmillan. Griggs was not given the volume on Kent, or he might have left us his own versions of the Palmer country; but it was through Griggs that Sutherland and Paul Drury, both in the etching class, came to know Palmer's work and spread the word.

I remember, on one of my sketching expeditions to the Shoreham Valley – this was before any of us knew of the Palmer connection – making notes of a splendid old barn. Later, comparing them with Palmer's drawings of the same landscape in the 1820s, I realised that I had unknowingly recorded the barn at

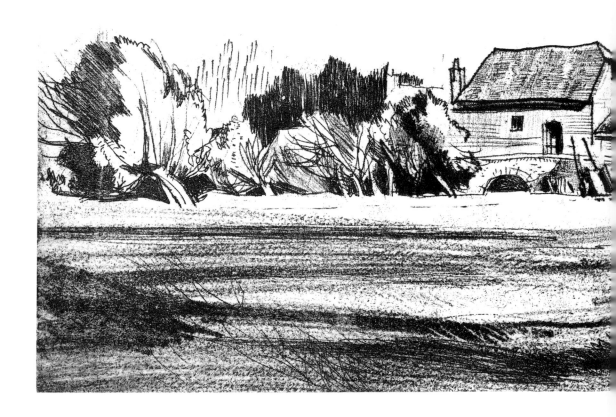

Sepham Farm, which appears in several of his drawings of the Shoreham period, still with its deeply thatched roof, massive doors and general appearance of having sat in those fields since time began. I was only just in time, as it turned out; within a year or two it had begun to collapse, and its present-day substitute is hardly worth a glance. Palmer, though not a topographical artist, used the components of the valley landscape, including its buildings, to express his almost sacramental feeling towards it. I was not the only youthful artist who, once Palmer's visionary genius was revealed, looked at his valley with different eyes. At the time, though, I was not looking with a *painter's* eyes – my instinct was that of a draughtsman and etcher. Palmer's paintings and drawings do have a strong linear quality which I and my friends recognised at once, and which, to a greater or lesser extent, left its mark on us all. Apart from him, we did not know of any major painter whose work was based on the technique we were being taught to master, the expression of line and form by graphic means alone.

We went back to Griggs, who was living deep in the Cotswolds for fear of contamination by the real world, with renewed interest in his Palmer-ish illustrations and drawings, in which no hint of the twentieth century was allowed to intrude. I cannot pretend that this pastoral intensity meant as much to me then as it was to later. I was already set on learning to paint, not merely draw. My heroes were such artists as John Arnesby-Brown and Alfred East, working in what could be loosely called a post-impressionist manner which is the opposite of the pastoral, semi-devotional mode that runs from early English stained glass

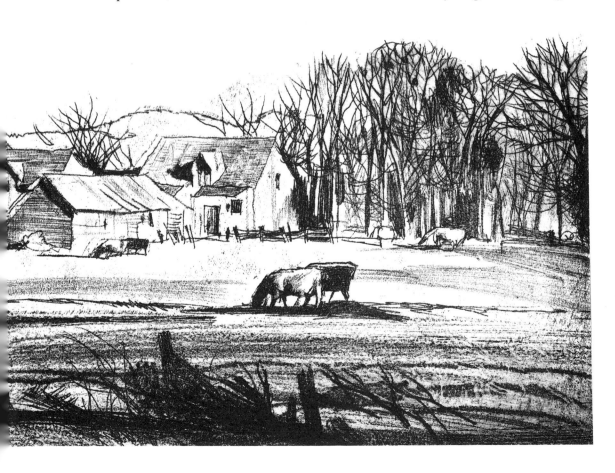

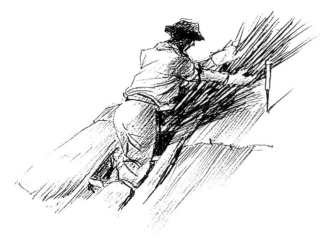

imagery through William Blake to Samuel Palmer, and which touches that disturbing character, Stanley Spencer. I recall his once telling me that, in the village he grew up in, religion was so essential a part of daily life that no one could get away from it, certainly not a budding artist. Cookham was sanctified by a simple belief that the Resurrection was an everyday event that was being re-enacted just down the road. What my fellow students and I saw in the Shoreham Valley was a staggeringly beautiful landscape, but I would not claim that it was a visionary experience.

I have sometimes wondered how it was that we could have been so unaware, as young hopefuls, of the long line of achievement in watercolour that stretches back two hundred years, to Alexander Cozens; Girtin; the equally young prodigy, Turner; Cotman and the Norwich painters. It takes an effort to realise that these names were never on our teachers' lips – Turner excepted, though only as a painter in oils – and that works by such early masters were nowhere to be seen. Those were the days when no one took watercolour seriously, except perhaps a handful of collectors who were rummaging happily for examples by our greatest artists, to be found for a few shillings each. Iolo Williams, who was one of these, and wrote a definitive book on the subject, claimed that he never, in a long life, paid more than a guinea for anything. In the Twenties, most English watercolours in the London salerooms were sold in multiple lots.

In this situation, as I have already remarked, one had to teach oneself, and perhaps it is that very fact that later enabled me to pass on my experience to others. The process was so slow that I had no difficulty in retracing my steps for the benefit of anyone who wanted to go the same way.

The main consideration for a professional painter who needs to make a living at it, as I do, is not to waste time and effort on subjects that would be unproductive. Nine-tenths of all the artists whose names first come to mind have been selective, as much for commercial reasons as for any other. And, of course, fashions and markets are changing all the time, and it would be insensitive not to respond in one's own way. For example, when I was at Goldsmiths' the idea of adding colour to an etching or original print would have been unthinkable. Today, in response to the public's familiarity with colour printing of all kinds, and of colour as the natural state of the world, as our eyes and television screens remind us all the time, printmakers no longer feel obliged to work only in black and white; though here I must make an exception of my friend and fellow student at Goldsmiths', Robin Tanner, whose pastoral etchings of the Wiltshire countryside are as gloriously black and white in 1987 as they were when we were twenty years old together. Again, original prints used to be small, as modest in scale as they were in subject. Today, at the print exhibitions at the Bankside Gallery, the walls are laden with fine coloured prints, some of them the size of a table top, competing on equal terms with watercolours and paintings following a complete change-round in the market.

I have found that most subjects can benefit from a little judicious rearrangement. I like the story of Monet, when he was a young nobody, putting on his only suit one morning, donning his top hat, and sauntering off to the Gare St. Lazare, where he introduced himself to the station-master as 'Monet, the painter'. He would like to paint the station-master's station, he announced. And would he get the firemen to stoke up the boilers, so as to generate a lot more steam? He got away with it, and the world got a marvellous painting. I have not gone so far, in setting up a promising subject, as that. But I make it a practice to re-order the components of a landscape, their relationships to one another, if by doing so I can enhance the inherent dignity of the whole. By 'dignity' I do not necessarily mean masses; details, too, contribute, such as a patch of weeds, the way a barn door hangs, an abandoned wagon.

One of the facts of life is that, when one's work begins to be noticed, other people are prompted to 'do a Hilder' themselves. I must say I feel ambivalent about it. It is agreeable to think that one has been able to help, and perhaps improve other people's skills. It is flattering for an artist to know that he has a following, and there is nothing unusual in that. It has happened throughout history, and a fairly senior painter who has been around long enough for his work to be widely familiar can expect it to happen to him, to a greater or lesser extent, as time goes by. That is as it should be. On the other hand, who is to say that derivative painting is a good thing? Andrew Wyeth, the American painter whose work so powerfully evokes the plain, puritan values of an older society than the one he actually lives in, has been so devotedly emulated and copied that he has gone so far as to say that his own art could turn out to be a disaster for American painting.

I hesitate to draw any parallels; but imitation and pastiche do not make good art. When I am conducting a class I try to steer them away from my own style and encourage them to develop their own. It would be a pity if all the 'wrong' Hilders were traced back to the artist himself! There is a story told of Picasso, when somebody turned up with a work of his and asked him to sign it, refusing point-blank to do so, saying it was a fake. 'But maître,' exclaimed someone else who was present at the time, 'I was here last summer when you painted that.' 'Oh yes,' Picasso said, 'I often paint my own fakes.'

Soon after my discharge from the Army Camouflage Corps in 1946 the idea occurred to us of looking for a large country house, which we would share with a couple of other families on a community basis, children, pets, nannies and all. We settled on a handsome eighteenth-century house with extensive grounds just south of Sevenoaks, called St Julian's. There I had a studio with a glorious view across the Weald, into which deer would stroll from Knole Park, just next door.

Out of the blue, in this period, came an opportunity for Edith and myself to collaborate on an ambitious project for Shell, for whom I had done poster work in the 1930s in their successful promotion campaign, using designs by prominent artists of the time. Edith had been at Goldsmiths' a couple of years behind me, a very good draughtsman (or should I say 'draughtsperson' these days?) with a rare talent for painting flowers. One day in 1953 I received a call from George Rainbird, one of the great innovators of the publishing business in this century,

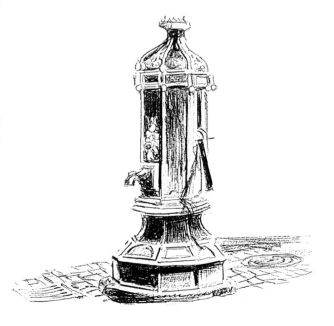

with an idea from Shell. He had come across a flower painter whom he thought highly of, and he asked if I would like to provide a series of background landscapes, into each of which this artist would introduce a particular study of wild flowers. Instead, I showed him some pictures by an artist whose style would merge perfectly with mine, with whom I would love to work, and who was a specialist in painting flowers: Edith, who else? He accepted at once.

The 'Flowers of the Countryside' series was to break new ground as a colour advertising campaign in which the picture, not the product, was the message. It taxed us to the limit of our skills. We had no guide-lines, no precedent. We had to organise twenty flowers of different sizes into a single background every time, all in scale and botanically exact – if they were not exactly right, we knew we would have thousands of knowledgeable nature-lovers on our backs the moment our pictures came off the press. The text was entrusted to Geoffrey Grigson, whose literary reputation was equalled by the respect in which he was held as a naturalist.

The enterprise dominated our lives. For eighteen months we talked, sketched and lived English wild flowers. Anticipating the public's response, Shell set up an office to deal with correspondence. Torrents of letters poured in and every one was answered. The advertising campaign amounted to the publication of 13 million plates, in a wide range of magazines from *Picture Post* to *Punch*, every month for a year. It was followed by a book, bringing all twelve plates and text together, which went into several editions. The experience has not put Edith off painting flowers; but these days she does so purely for our enjoyment.

It was in those years, and throughout the 1960s, that Rowland Hilder cards began to be seen in such numbers on people's mantelpieces. Later, with my father's health failing, we joined forces with the printing firm of Royles. I was able, at last, to devote more time to painting; not before time, you might think, since I was by then nearly sixty. But my best years were still to come.

One of the many pleasures Edith and I share is visiting the wide, wild seascape off the east coast, where the River Swale and the creeks offer wonderful sailing. There, over the years, our son Anthony has grown into a seasoned yachtsman as well as advancing his professional talent as a marine artist. He spends all the time he can spare in sailing his 42-foot ocean cruiser, *Enigma*, and I sometimes join him as relief helmsman.

For a painter, life is never short of challenges. When, in the autumn of 1985, I was offered an exhibition at the Woodlands Gallery, Greenwich, with its handsome rooms and generous spaces for hanging, I saw it as an opportunity to develop my own watercolour art on a full scale. Many members of the public who visited the exhibition told me of their pleasurable surprise at seeing the originals of works which they had previously known only from much-reduced reproductions. Others that I have in mind will take the process further. Now, I enjoy a rare privilege. I paint as I please.

TIME AND PLACE

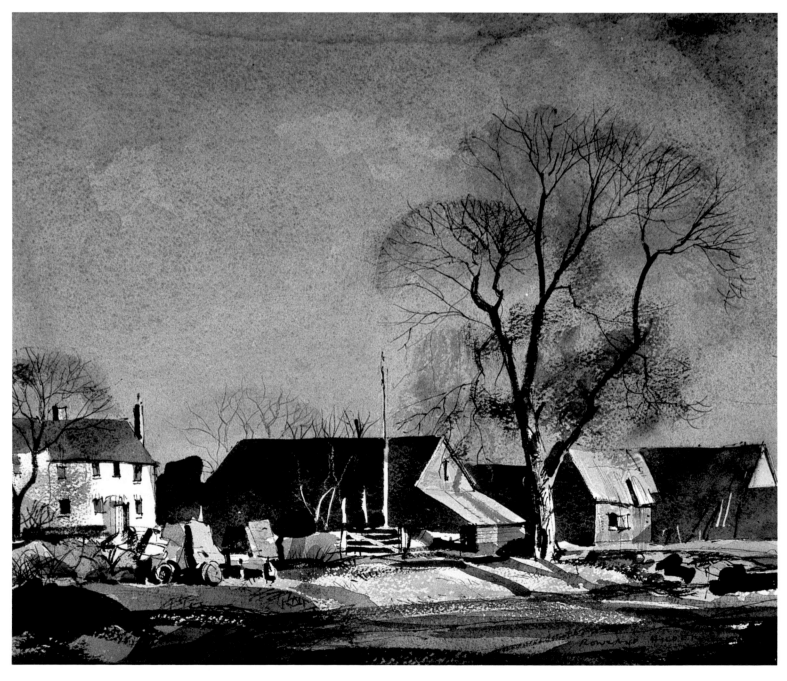

NORFOLK FARM

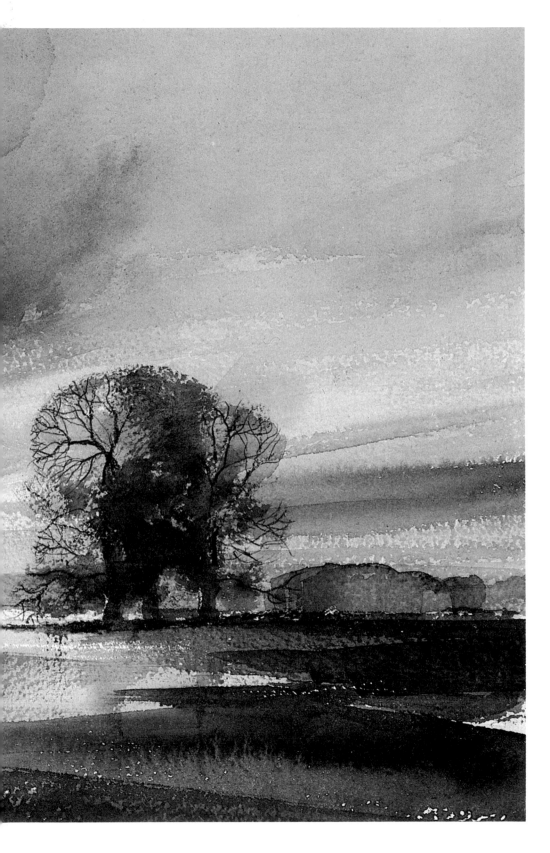

'It is not always my purpose
to sit down and paint literally
what my eyes tell me is there in
front of me, but to search for the
essence of the time and place.'

SEPTEMBER DAWN

19

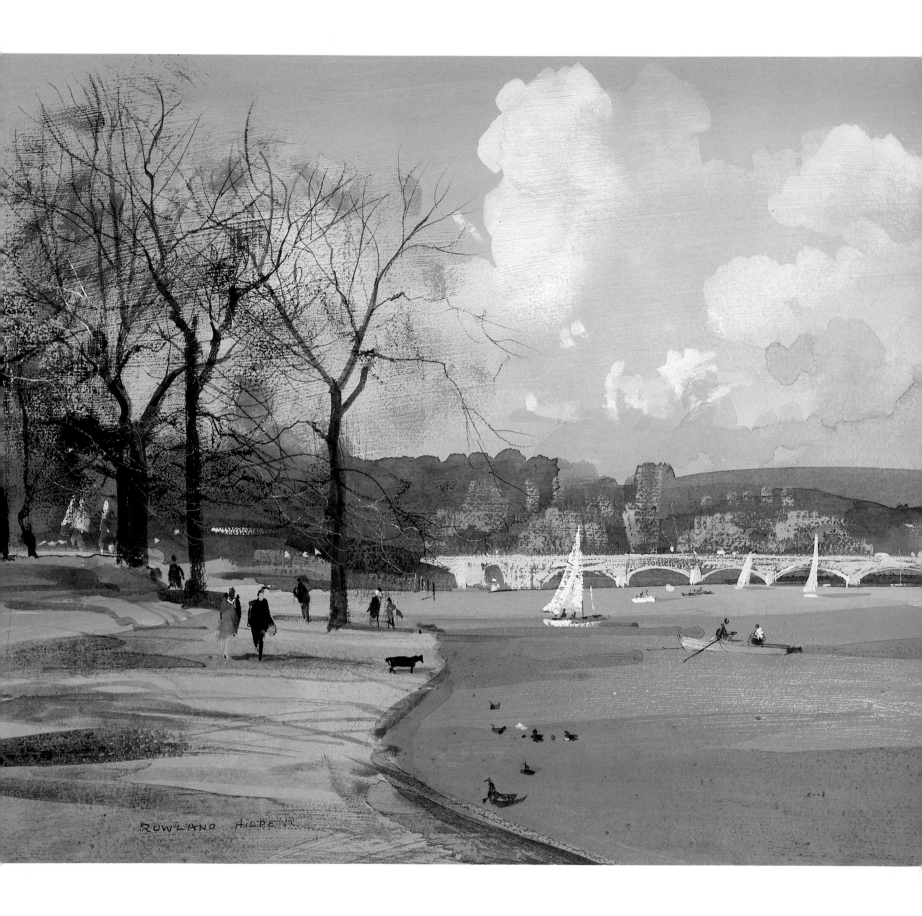

ROWLAND HILDER

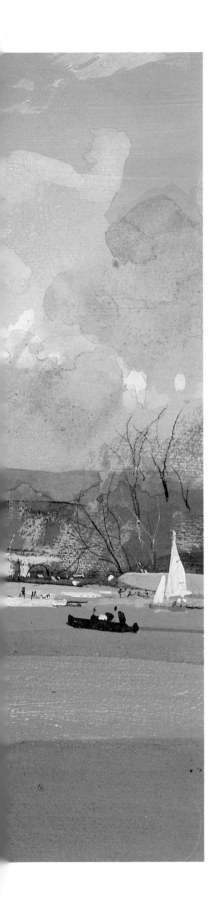

THE SERPENTINE, HYDE PARK

It gets its name from its shape rather than from anything slithery that might be lurking in it. Even so, most visitors prefer walking round its perimeter to chancing its sparkling waters.

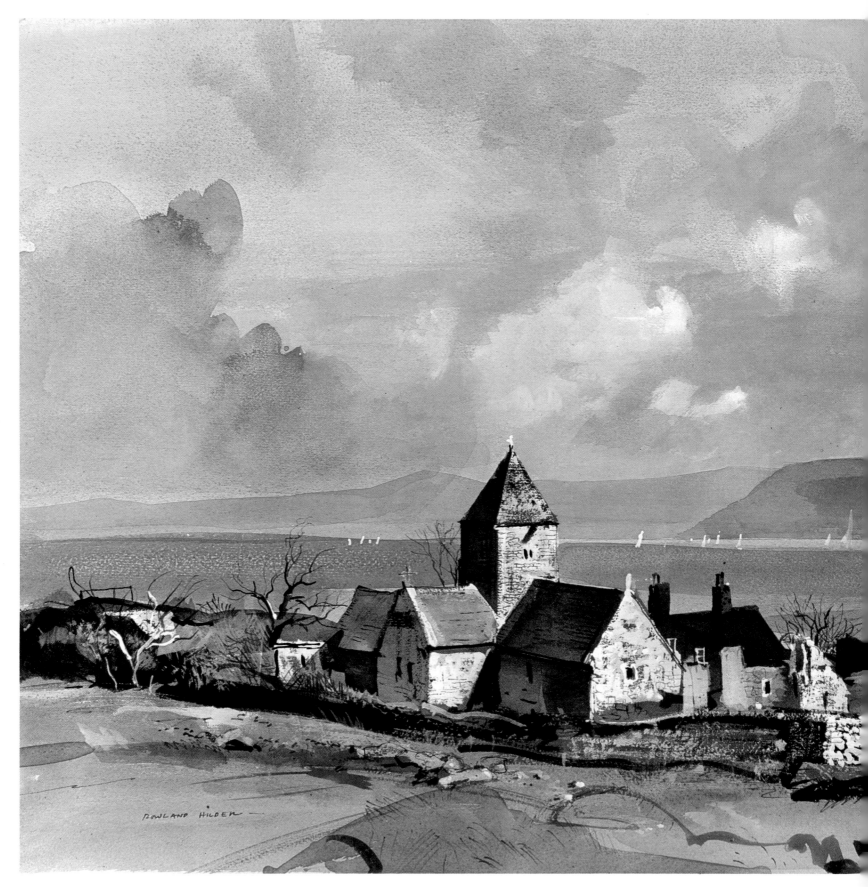

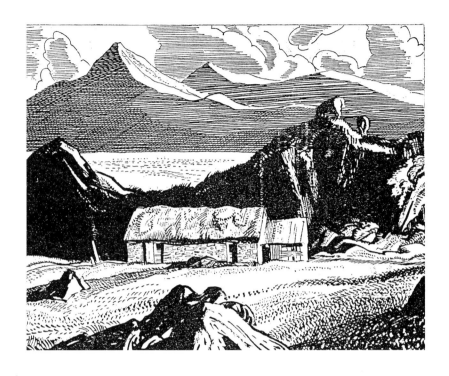

PENMON PRIORY, ISLE OF ANGLESEY

The tiny church and dovecote are Norman. The view across the Bay of
Conway to the Snowdon range cannot have changed in a thousand years.

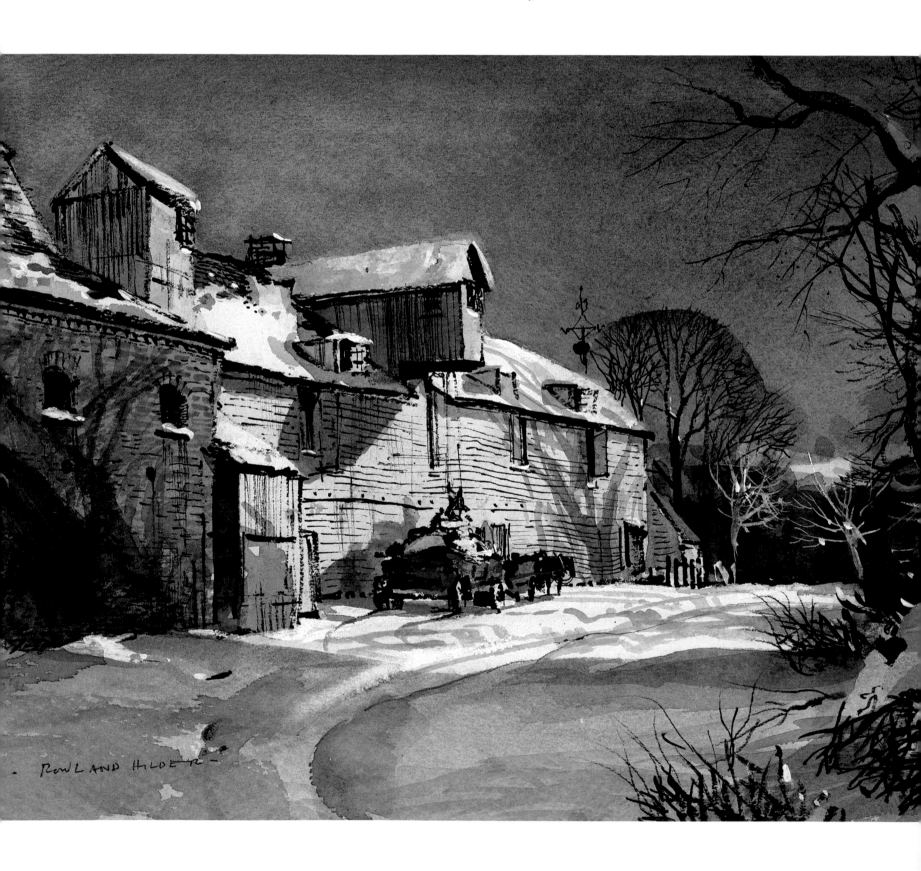

ROWLAND HILDER

24

MALTINGS IN EAST ANGLIA

Many old villages were working communities into modern times. Mills and maltings have survived in Suffolk and Norfolk, mostly now converted to what estate agents describe as 'character' homes.

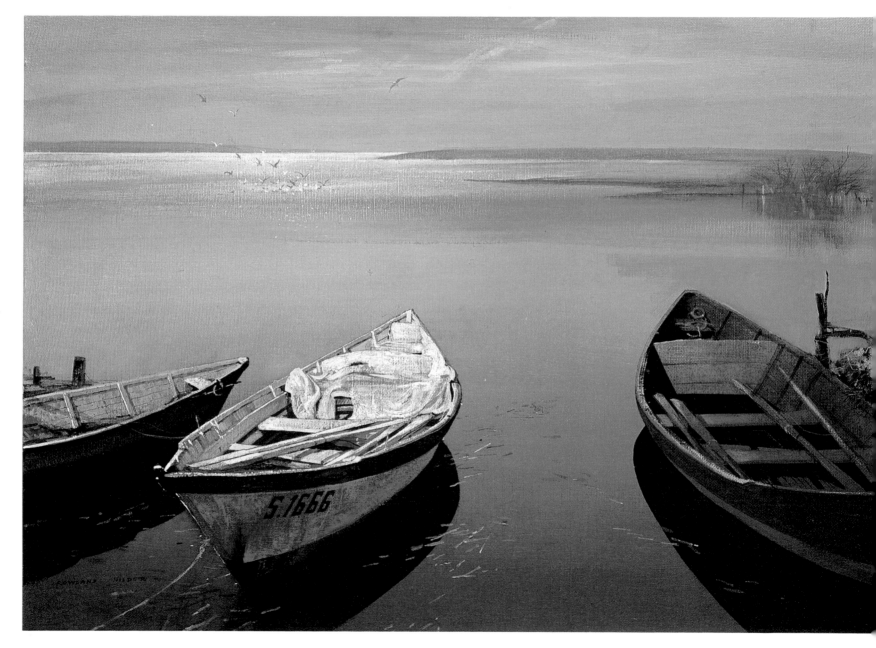

FISHING BOATS ON THE CAMARGUE

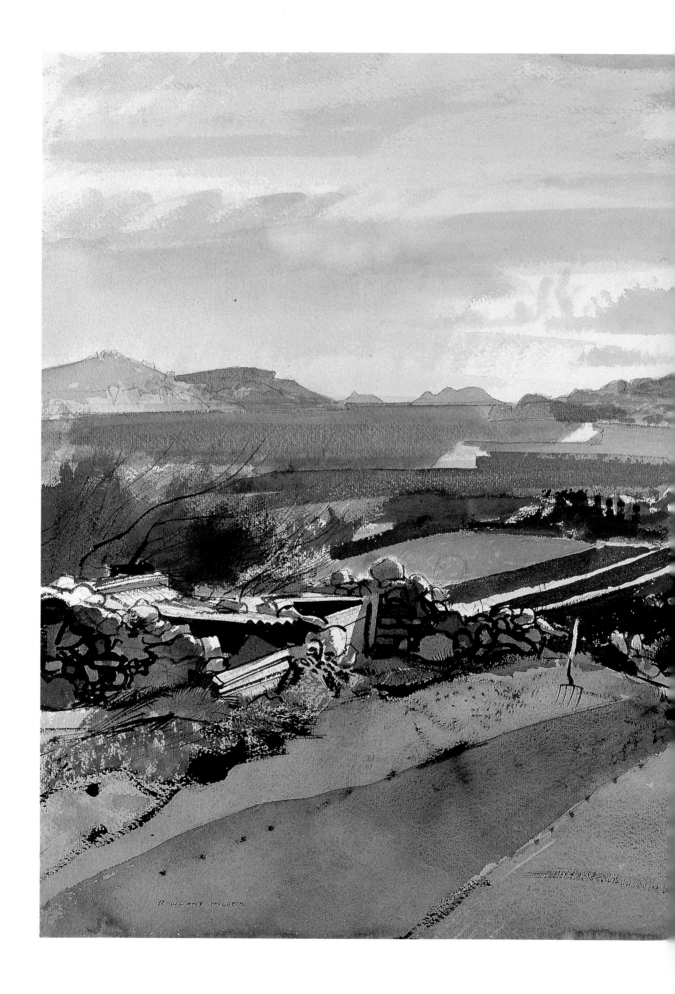

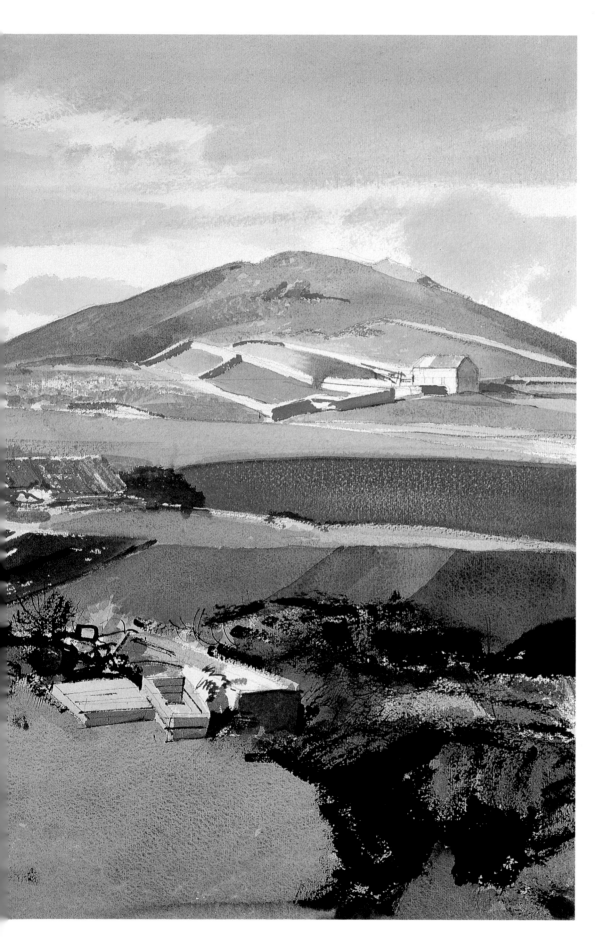

BRYHER, ISLES OF SCILLY

It is one of the relatively untrodden islets off the main archipelago of granite rocks, a Cornish outcrop in the sea. They grow daffodils here, ahead of the mainland's Spring.

LIMEHOUSE REACH (*overleaf*)

Due south from the Regents Canal system, Limehouse Reach is the last stage of a great loop that creates the peninsula known as the Isle of Dogs. Originally named after its lime kilns, nearby Limehouse has a history reaching back to 1380, when the first habitation for lime-burners was built on this bend of London's river. Decking the scene as it would have looked at the turn of the century seems a justifiable liberty on this time-worn spot.

27

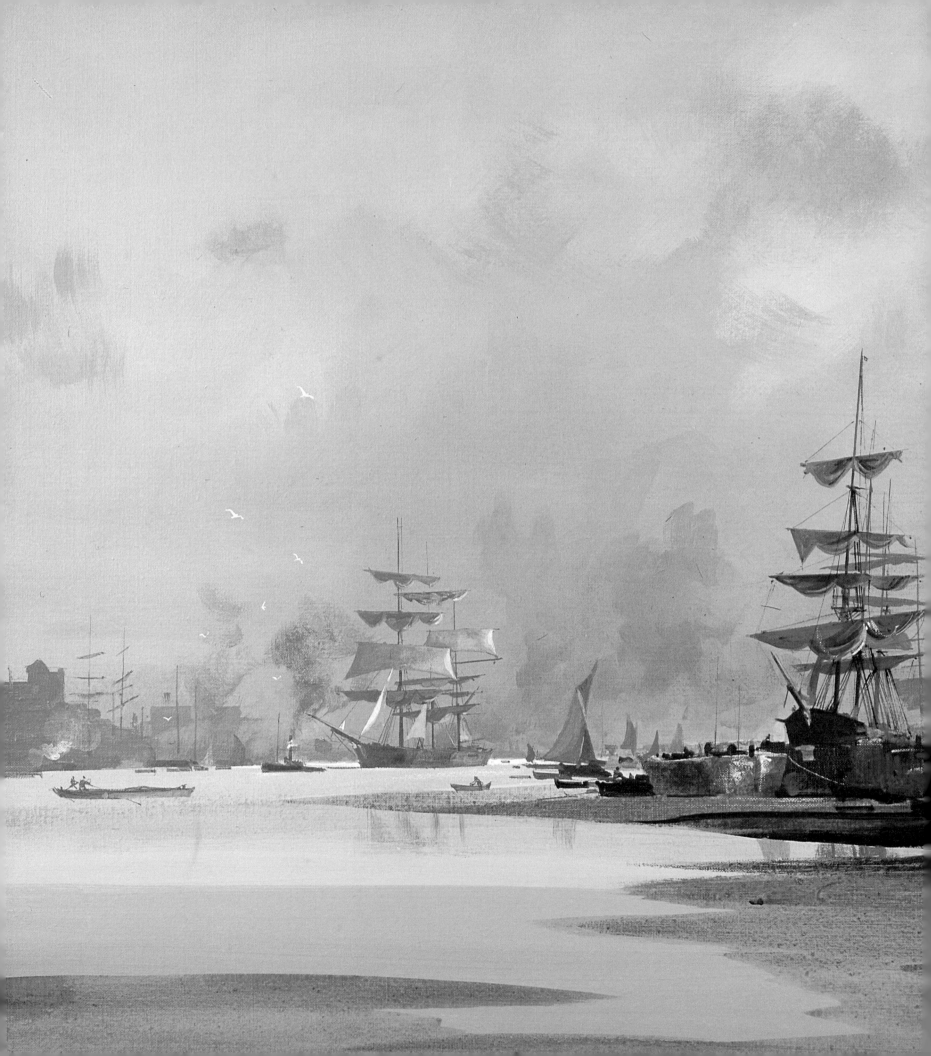

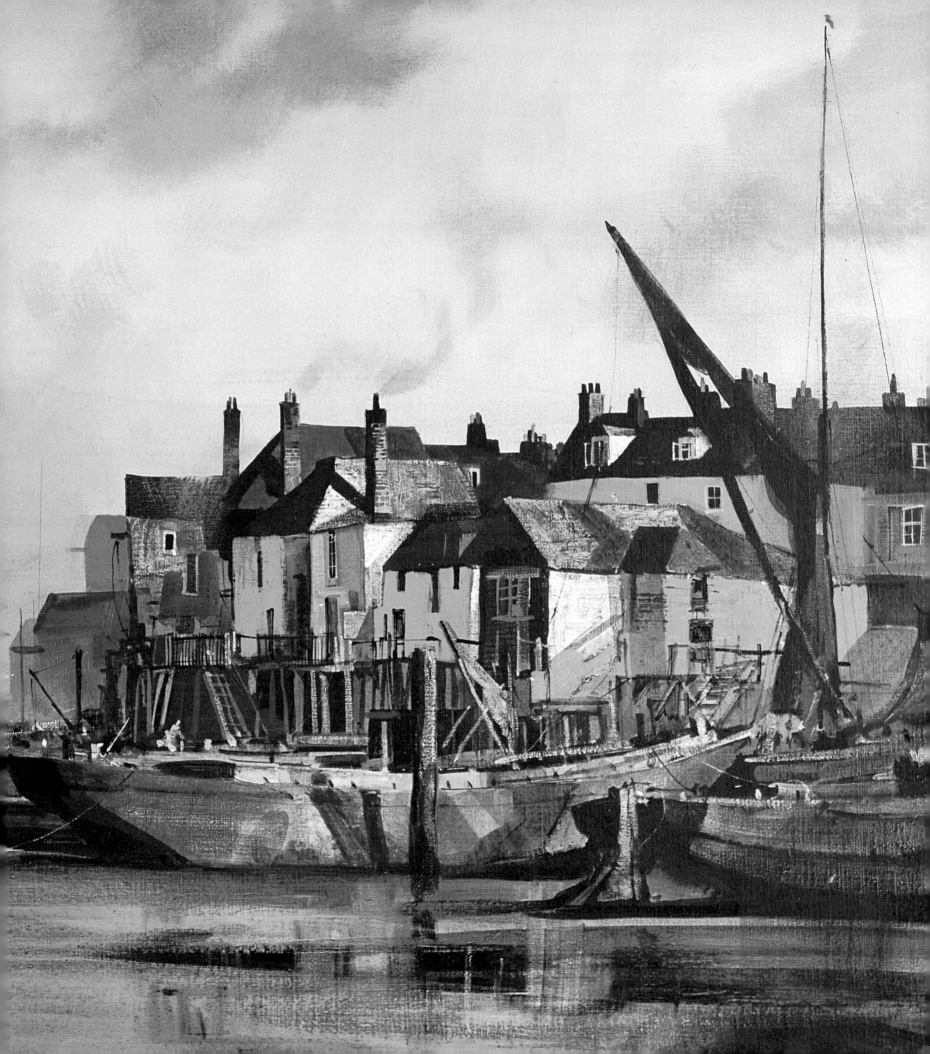

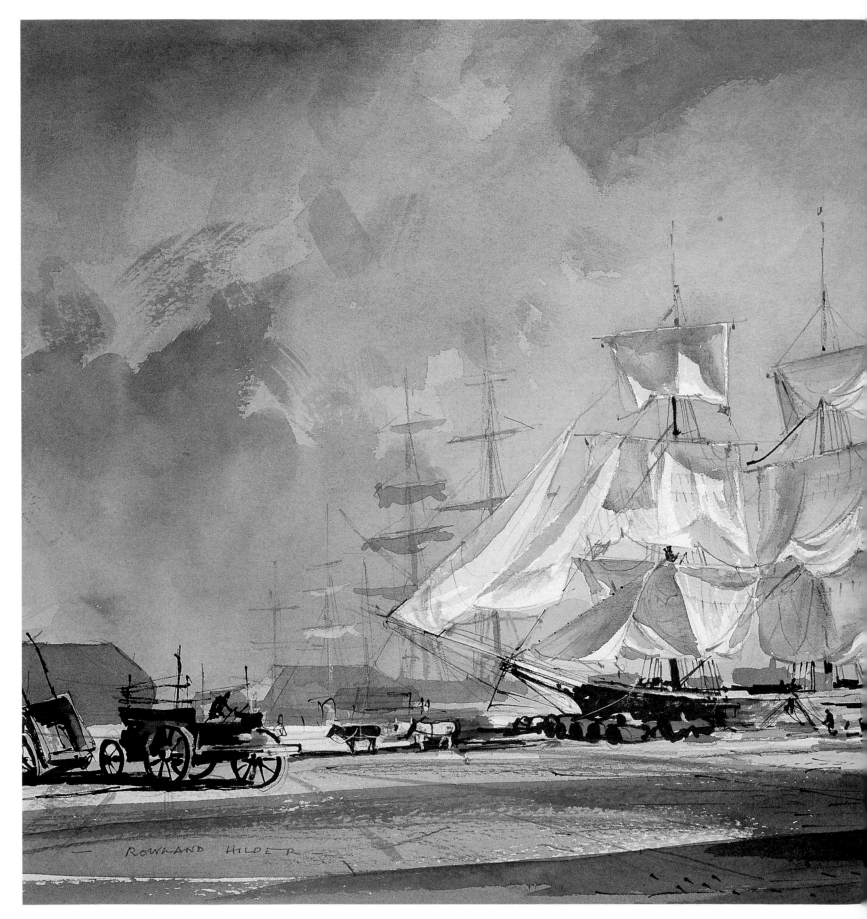

ROWLAND HILDER

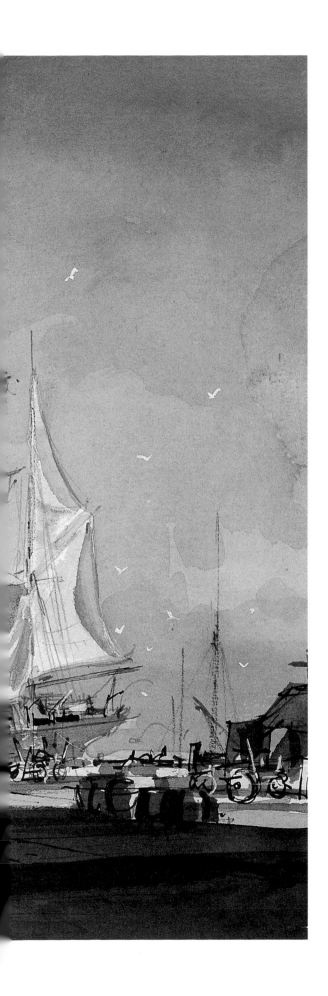

'I could not stop drawing it all: tugs, colliers, shipboard tackle, amazing rigging, furled sails, hooters, sirens, men rolling barrels, the tang of tar and the creeping promise of the sea.'

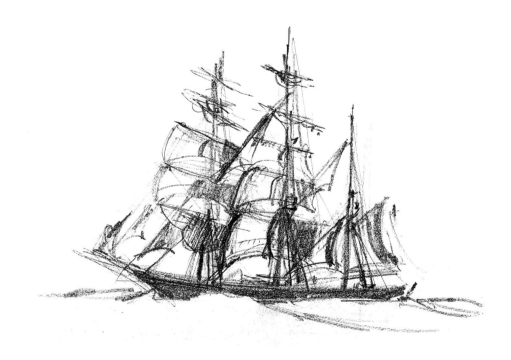

IN THE DAYS OF SAIL

All this is within the memory of people who were born at the turn of the century. To have glimpsed it, even in one's early childhood, is one of the benefits of age.

VISIONS FROM VENICE

Any painter who gets out his brushes on such a spot feels the presence of greater artists who have been there before him. Even on a day when it seems to be bathed in London weather, the light and mysticism are undiminished.

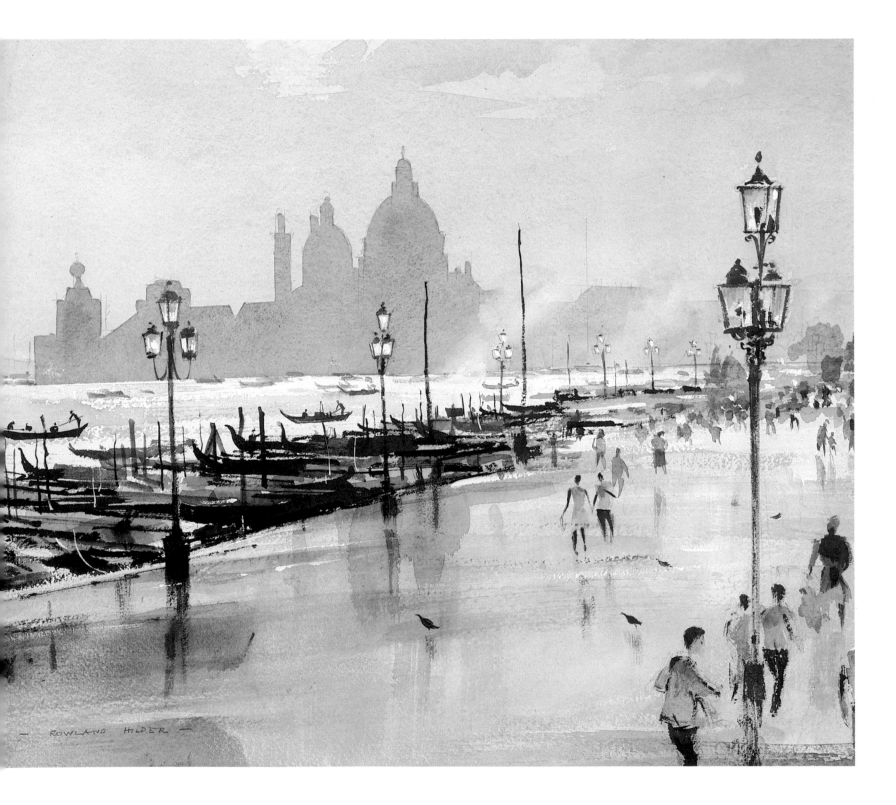

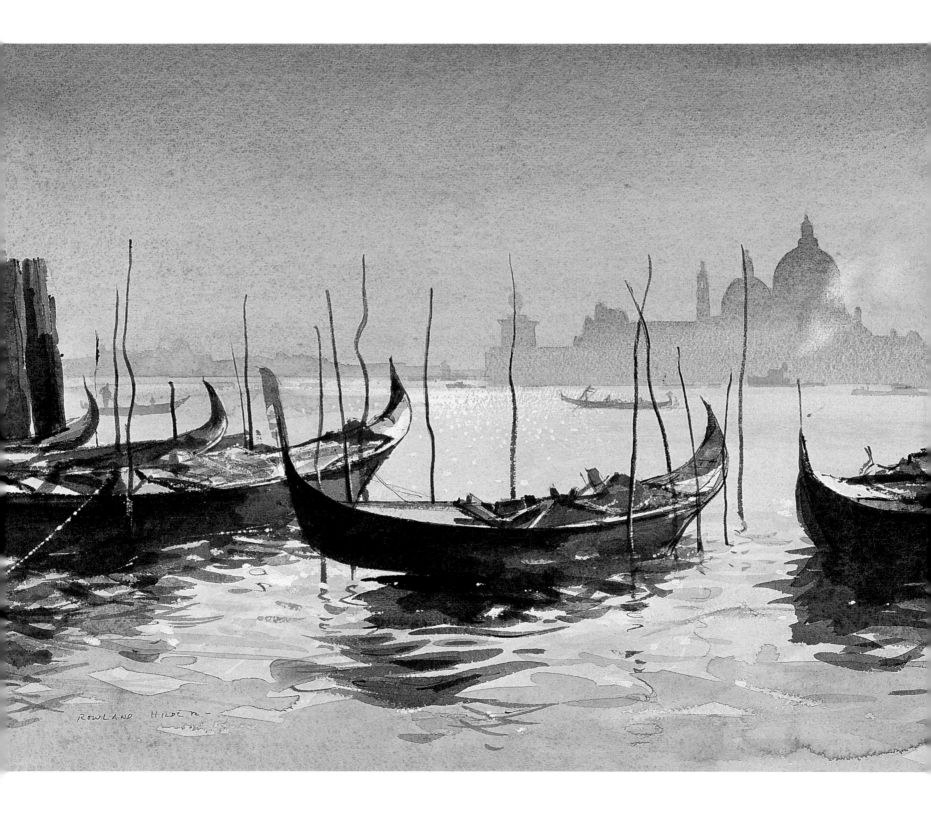

ROWLAND HILDER

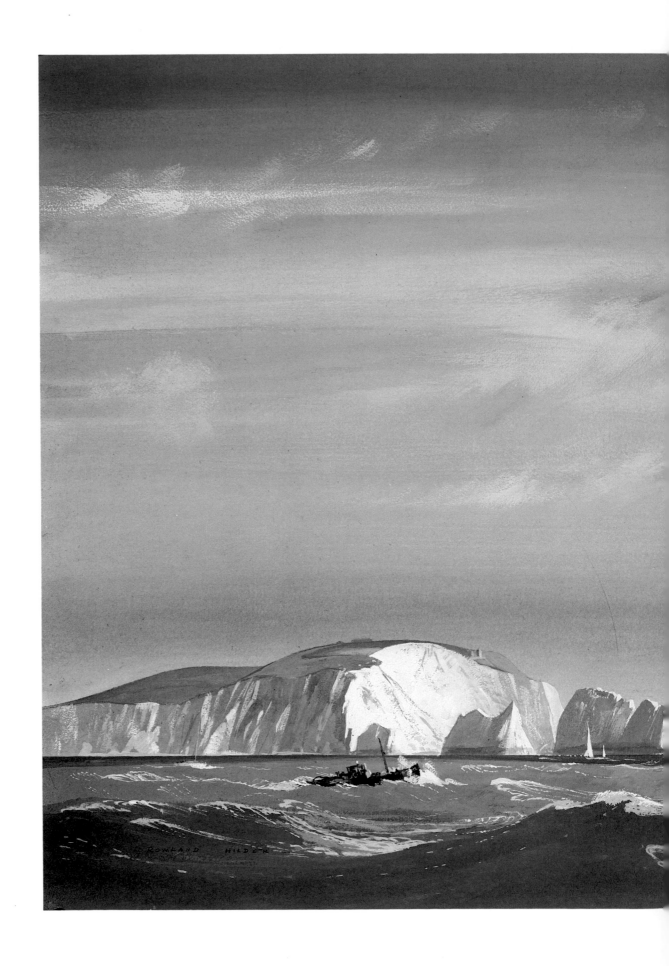

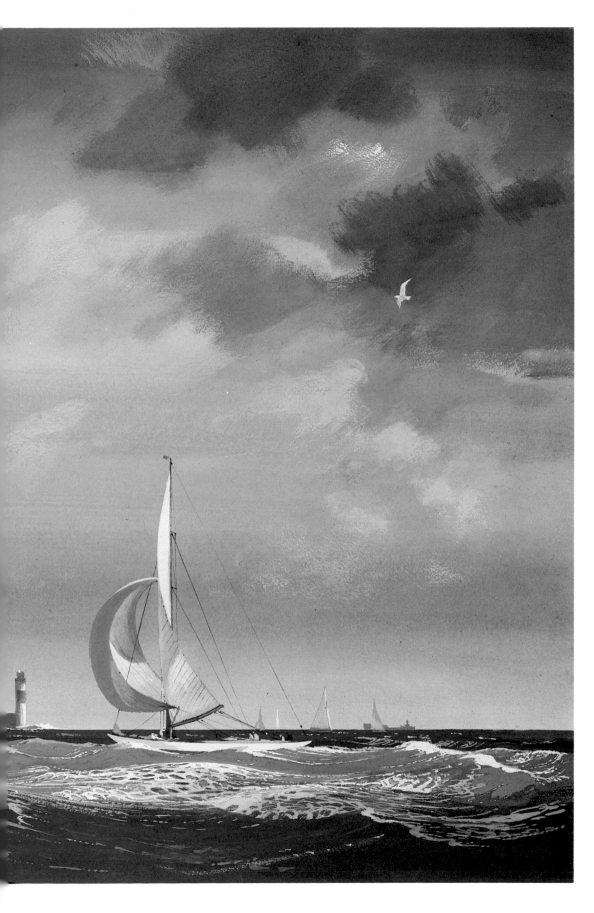

THE NEEDLES

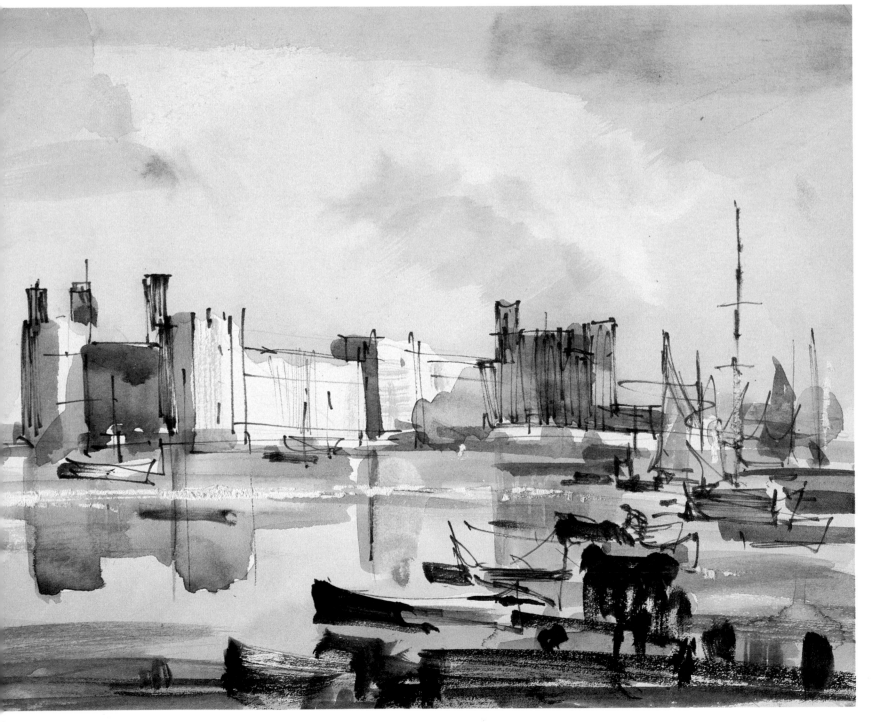

CAERNARVON CASTLE

TOWN AND AROUND

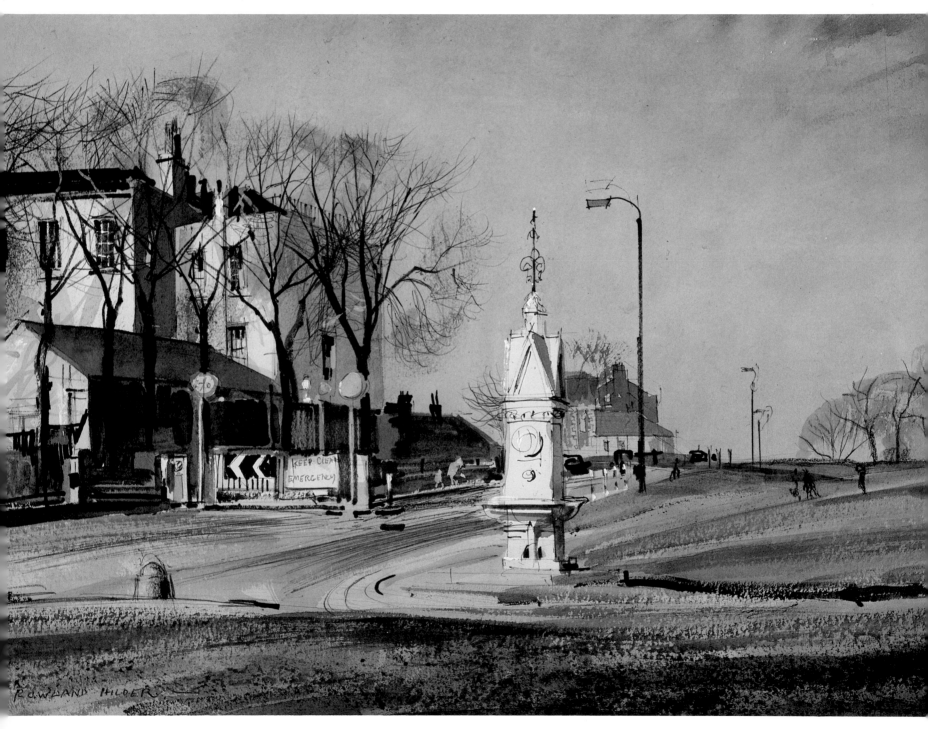

BLACKHEATH FROM TRANQUIL VALE

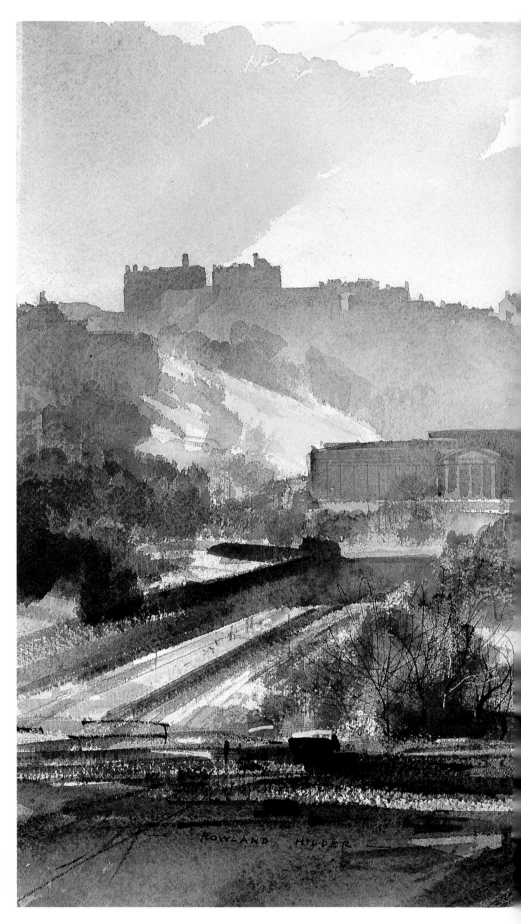

PRINCES STREET, EDINBURGH

The proud heart of Scotland's capital city, repository of idealism and clear thinking since the Age of Reason, and still a cultural force in a disbelieving world.

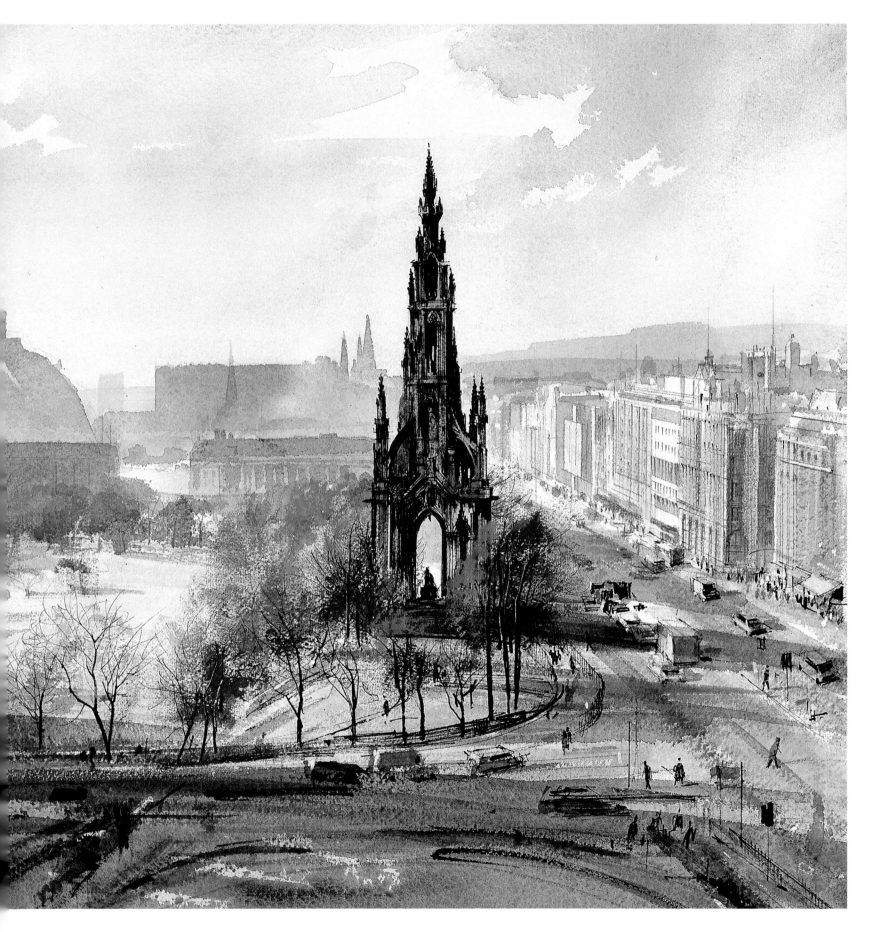

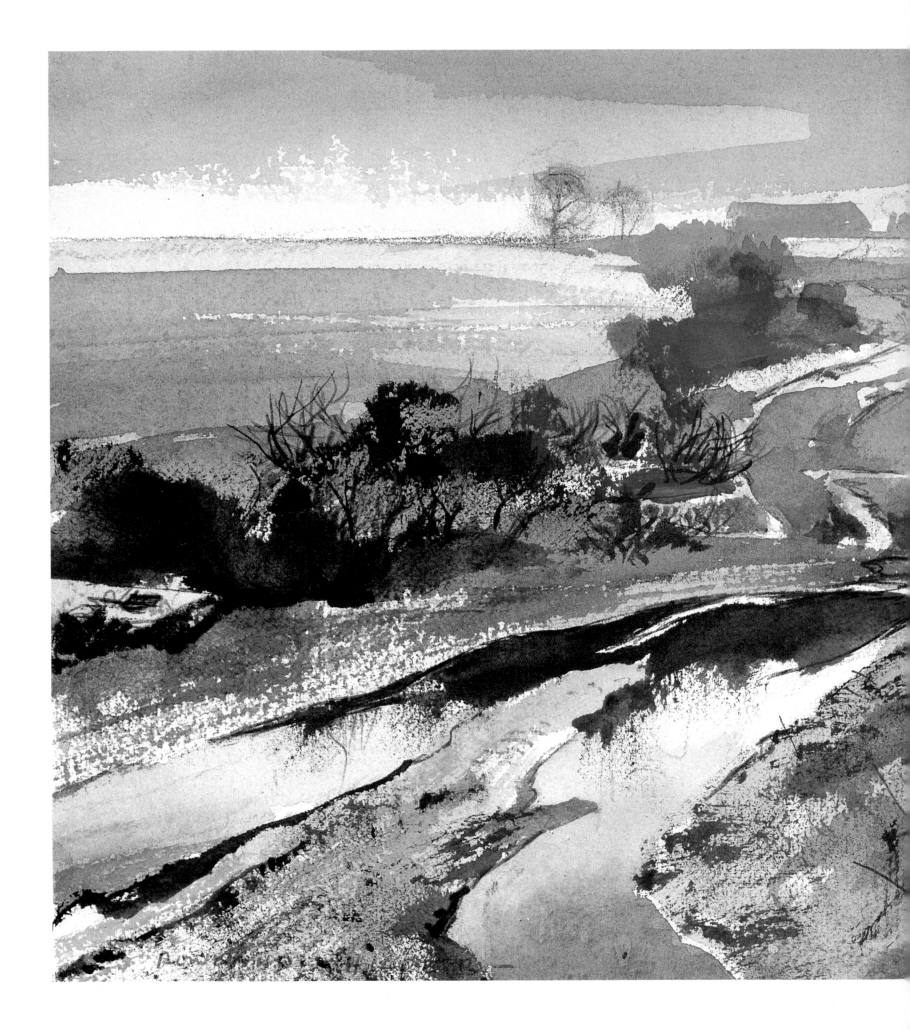

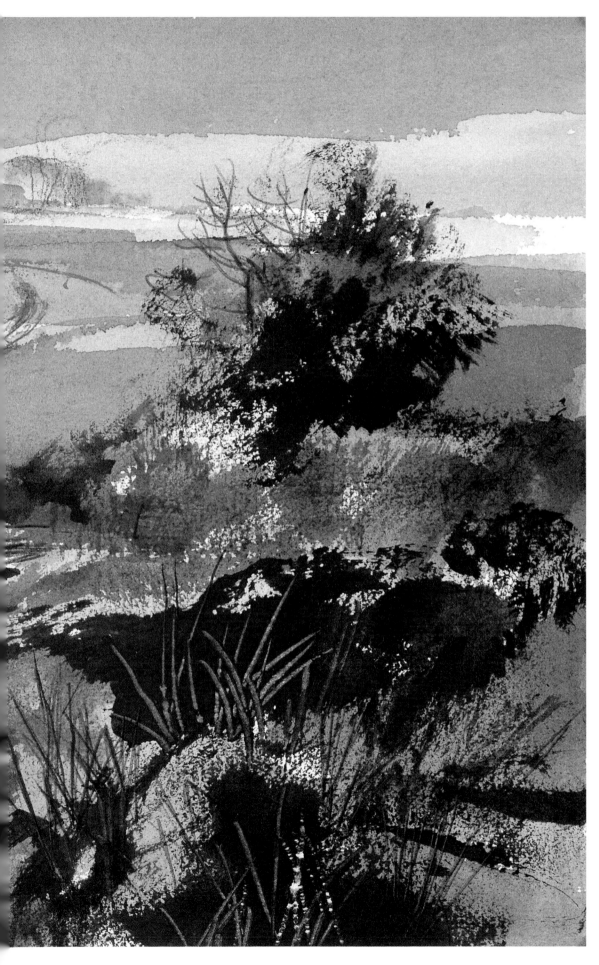

WAYSIDE LANDSCAPE,
KENT

41

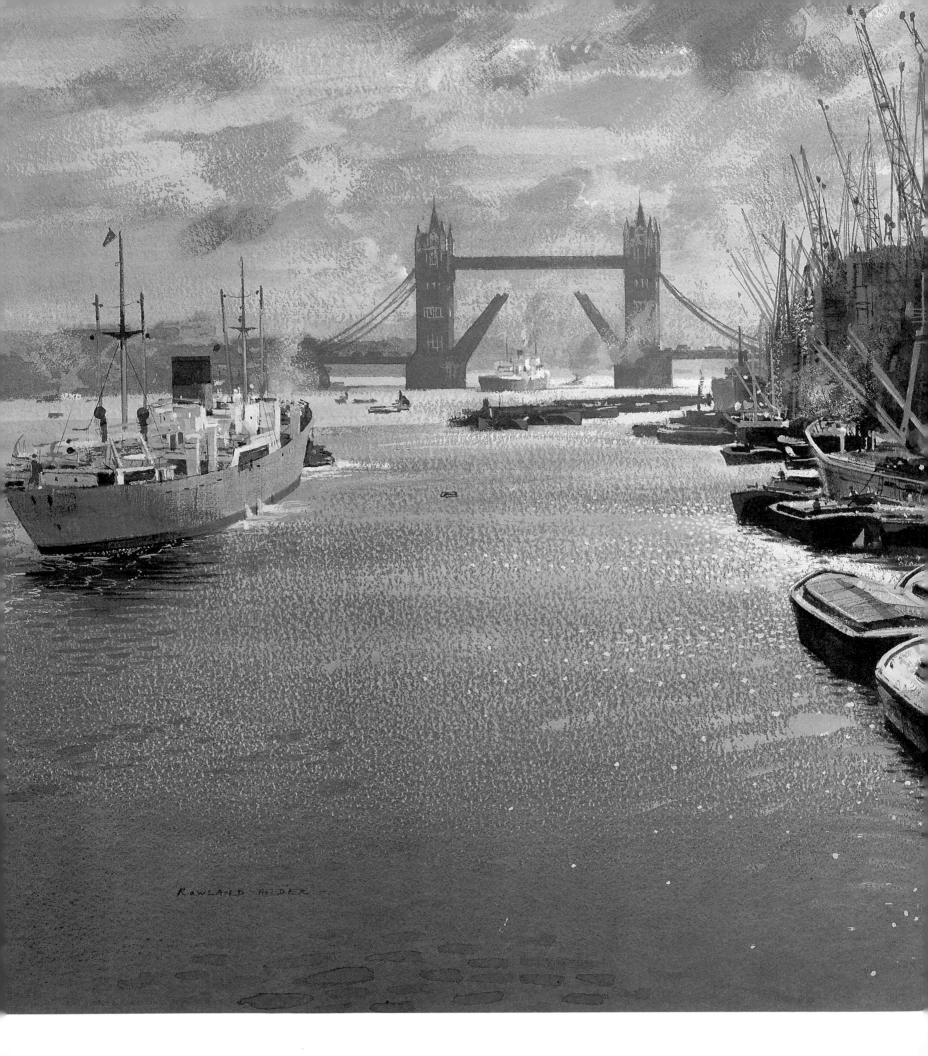

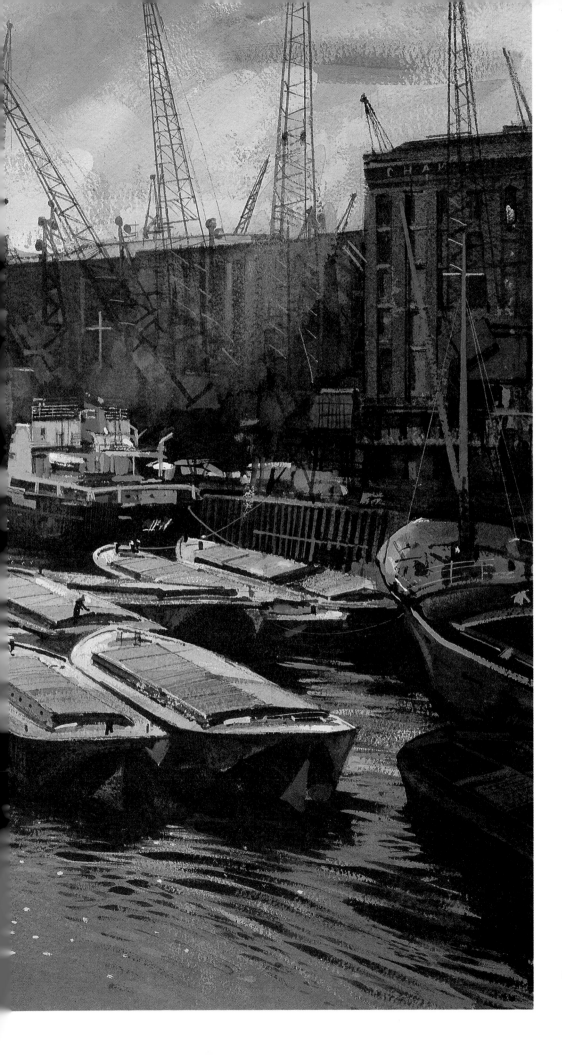

OLD THAMES AT TOWER BRIDGE

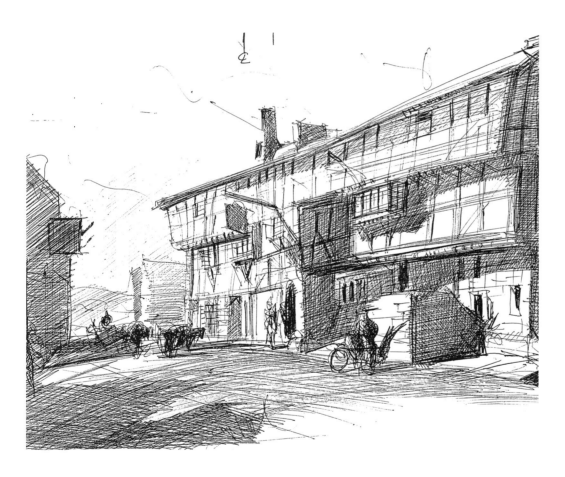

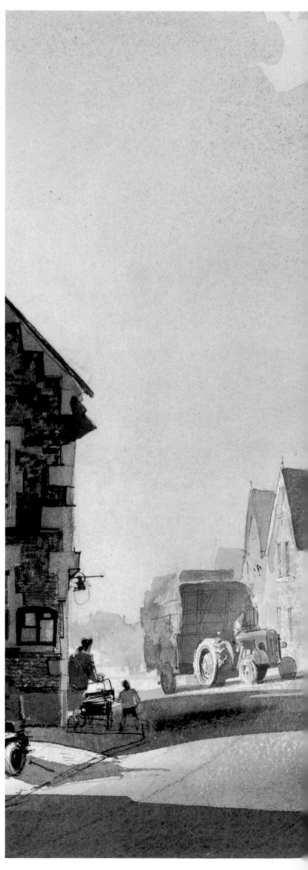

GEORGE INN, NORTON ST. PHILIP, SOMERSET

The epitome of the old English hostelry, built in 1397 for the Carthusian Priory of Hinton both as a storehouse for their wool and as accommodation for visitors to the market and cloth fair. The Duke of Monmouth took refuge here after the Battle of Sedgmore, and narrowly escaped with his life.

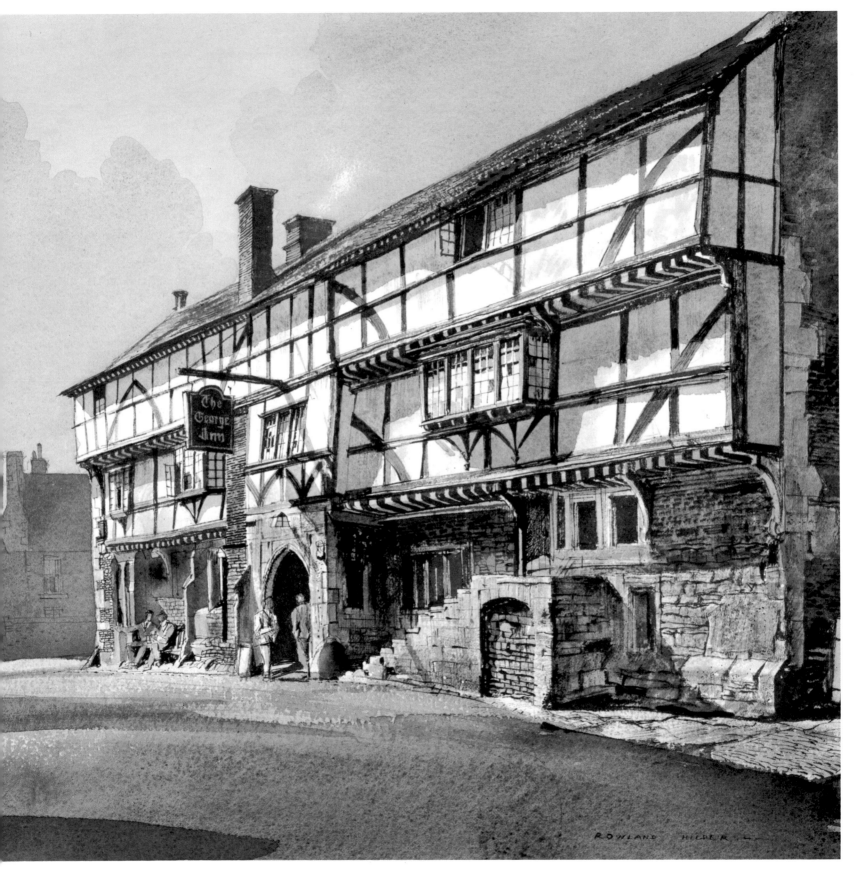

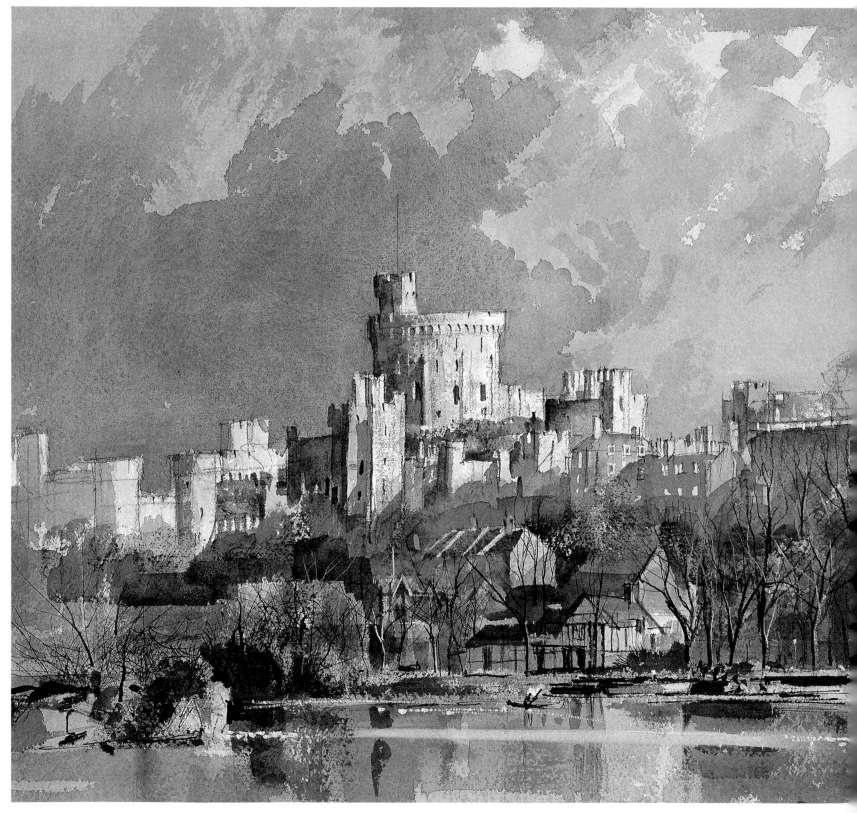

46

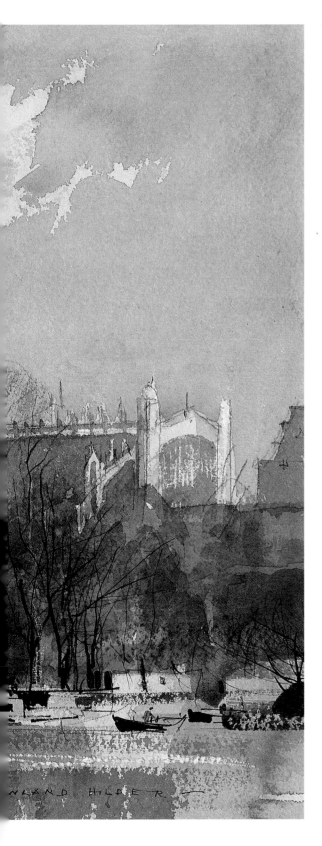

WINDSOR CASTLE

From the outside, the royal residence looks rather different from early pictures of it. Most of the exterior is nineteenth century, the Round Tower is much higher than Henry II's original, and various turrets have grown a few feet as a result of the Gothic revival in Victorian times. William the Conqueror, who started it in 1078, would recognise the motte-and-bailey layout.

(*Overleaf*) BICTON MILL, NEAR FORDINGBRIDGE, DORSET

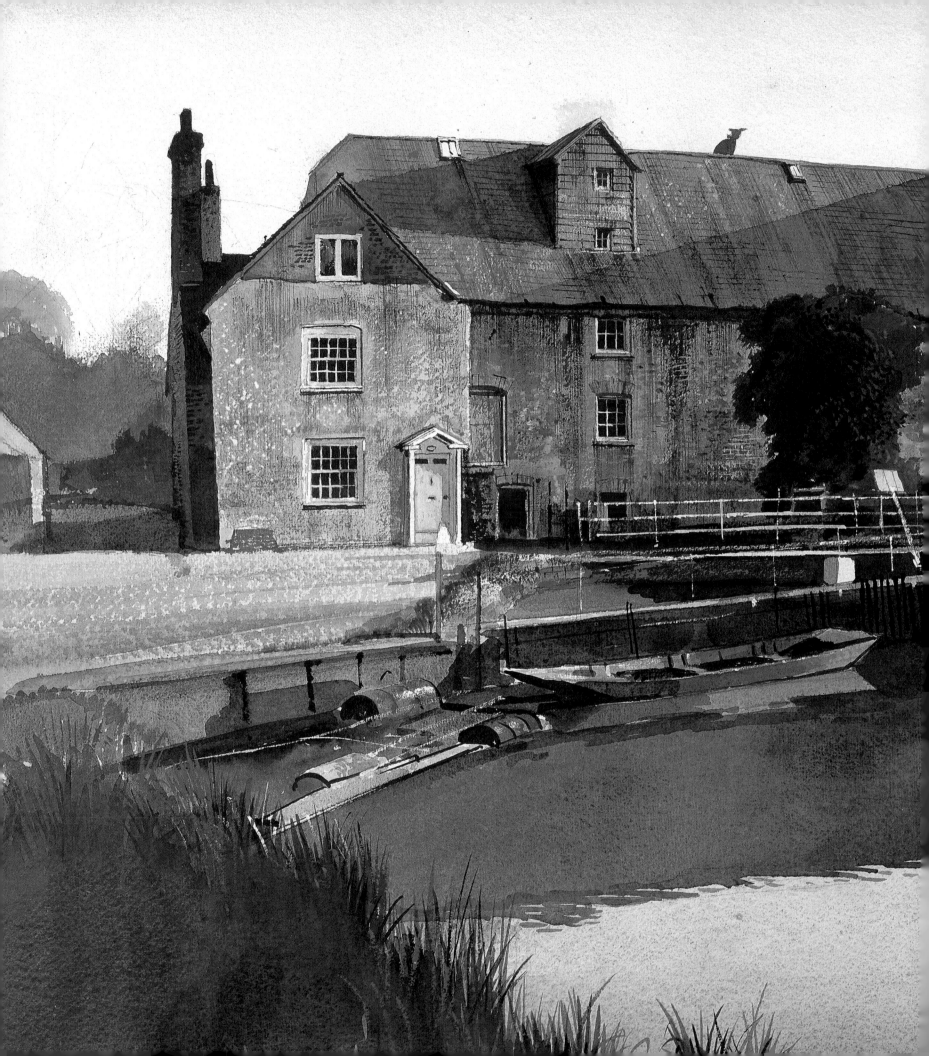

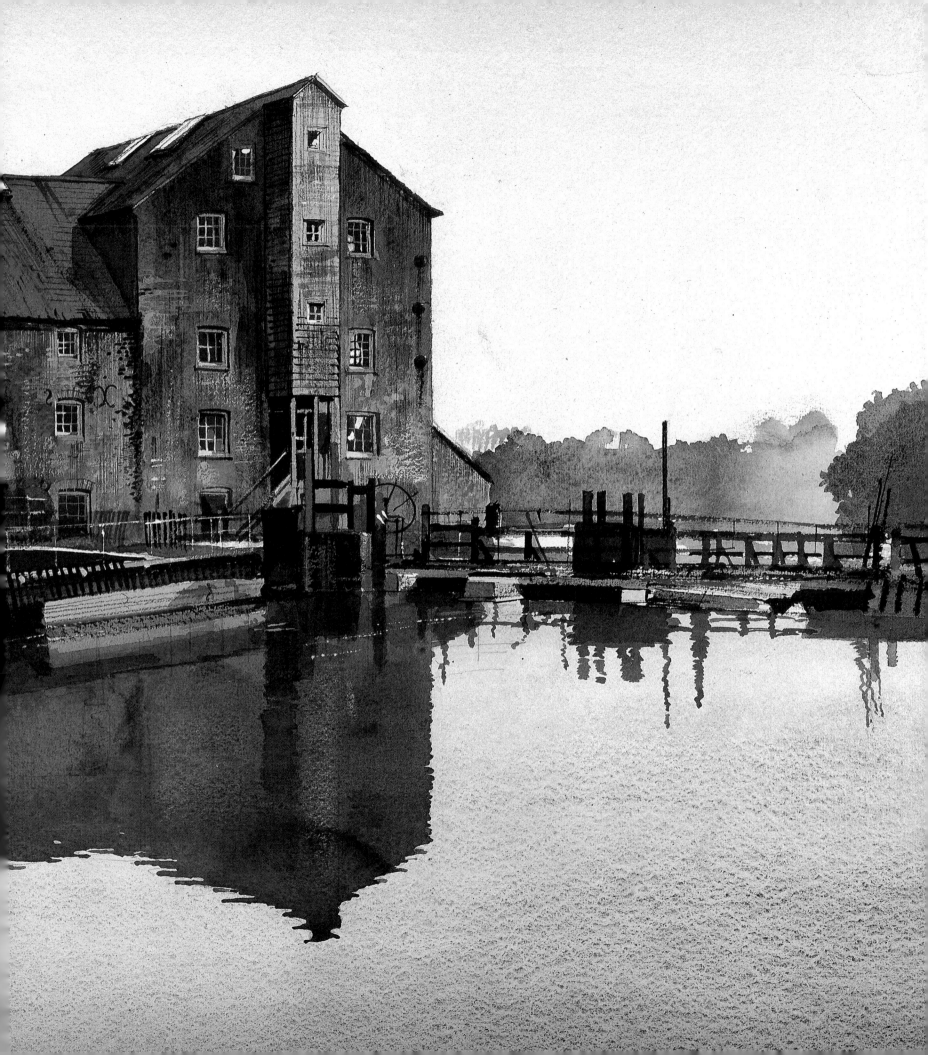

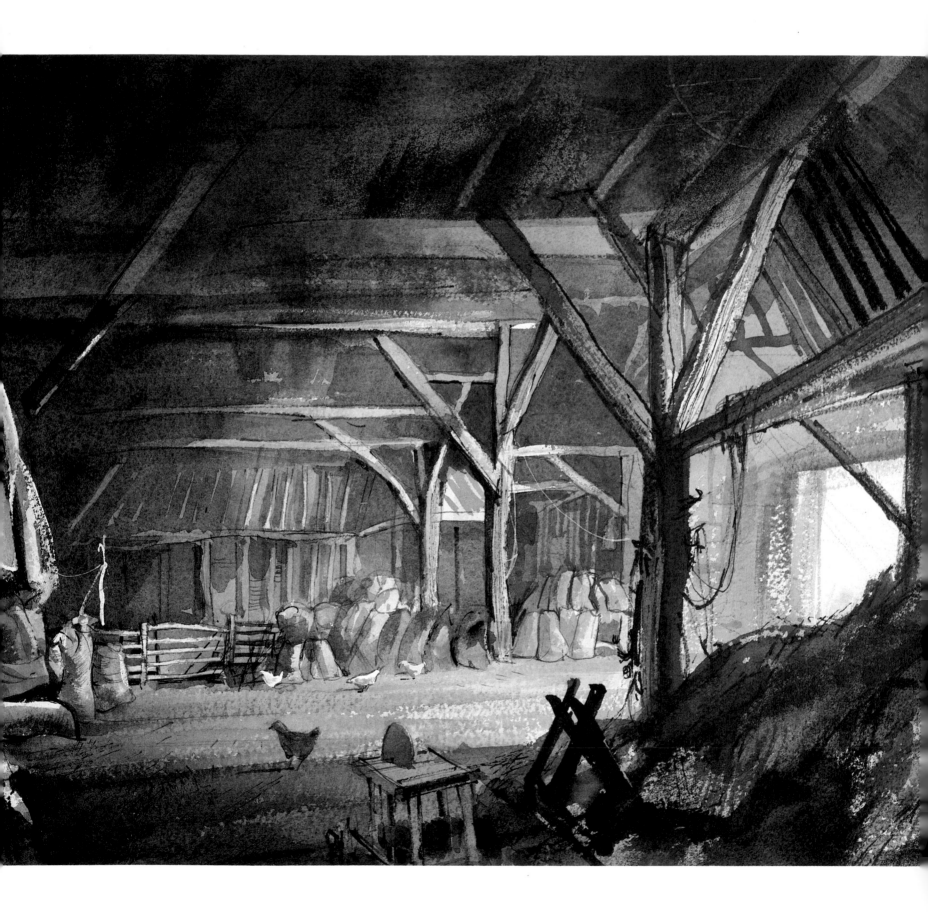

TITHE BARN

In the days when the Church had a legal claim to one-tenth of parishioners' grain, the local parson would store his tithe, or tenth, in a barn set aside for the purpose. The name lives on, though the custom does not.

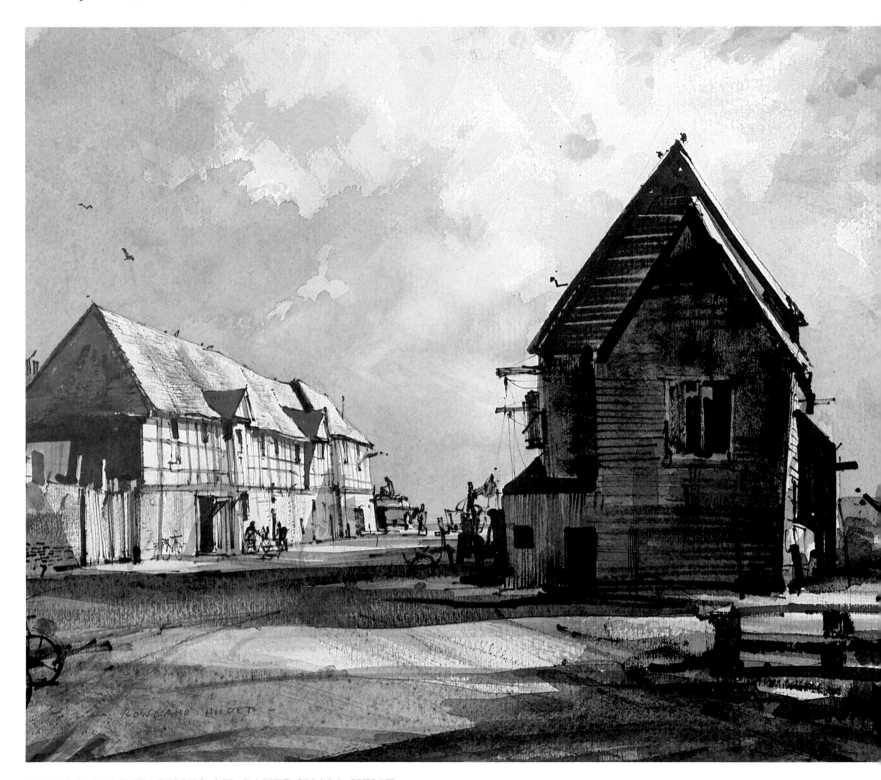

TUDOR WAREHOUSES AT FAVERSHAM, KENT

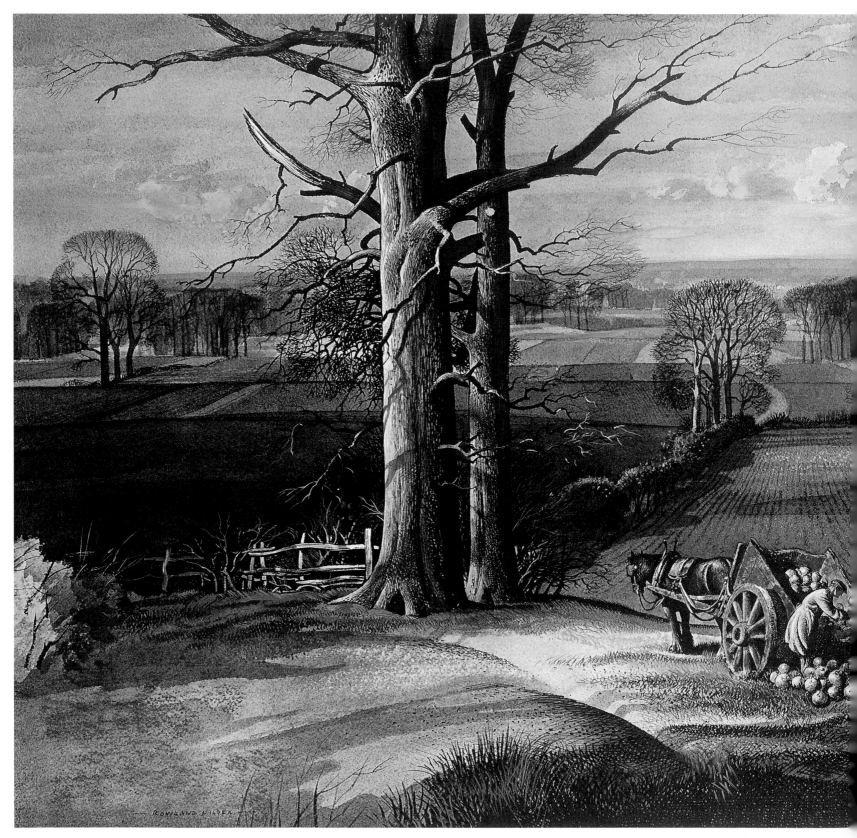

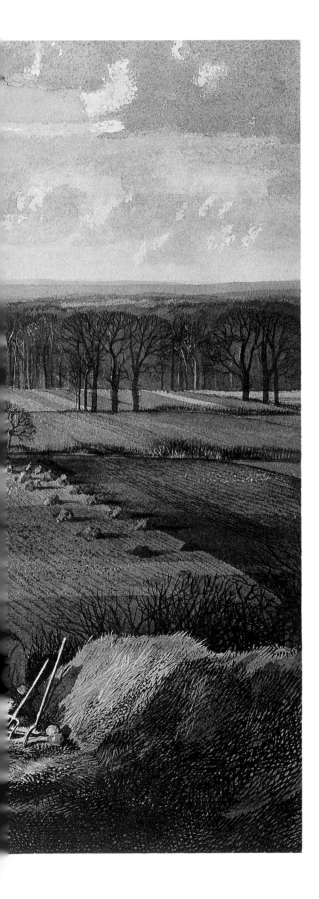

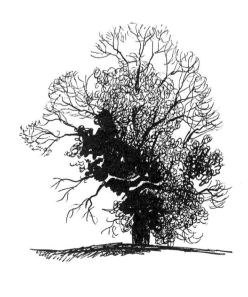

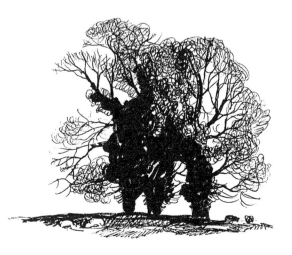

MORNING SUNSHINE

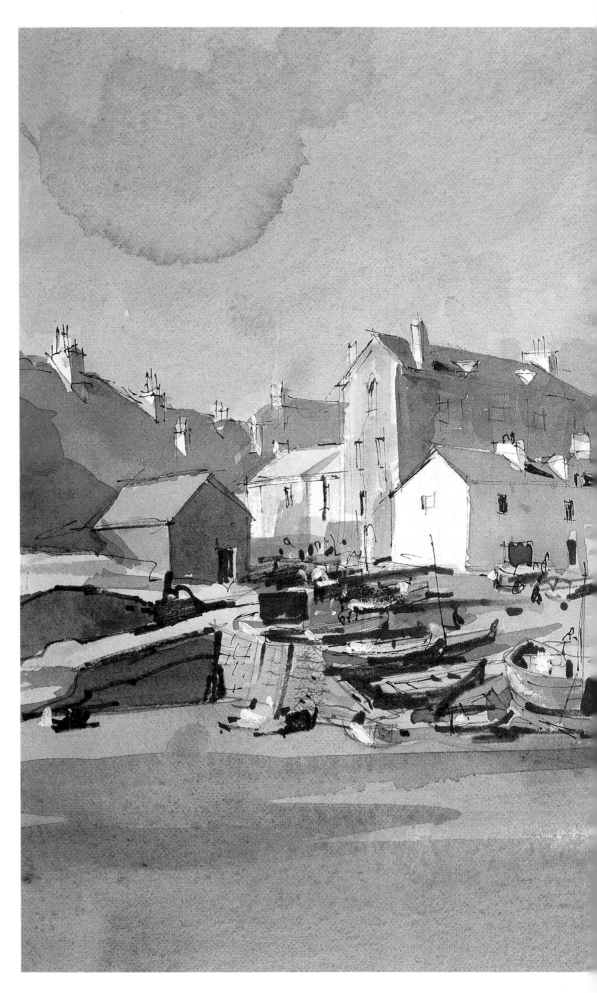

54　NEW QUAY, DYFED, WALES

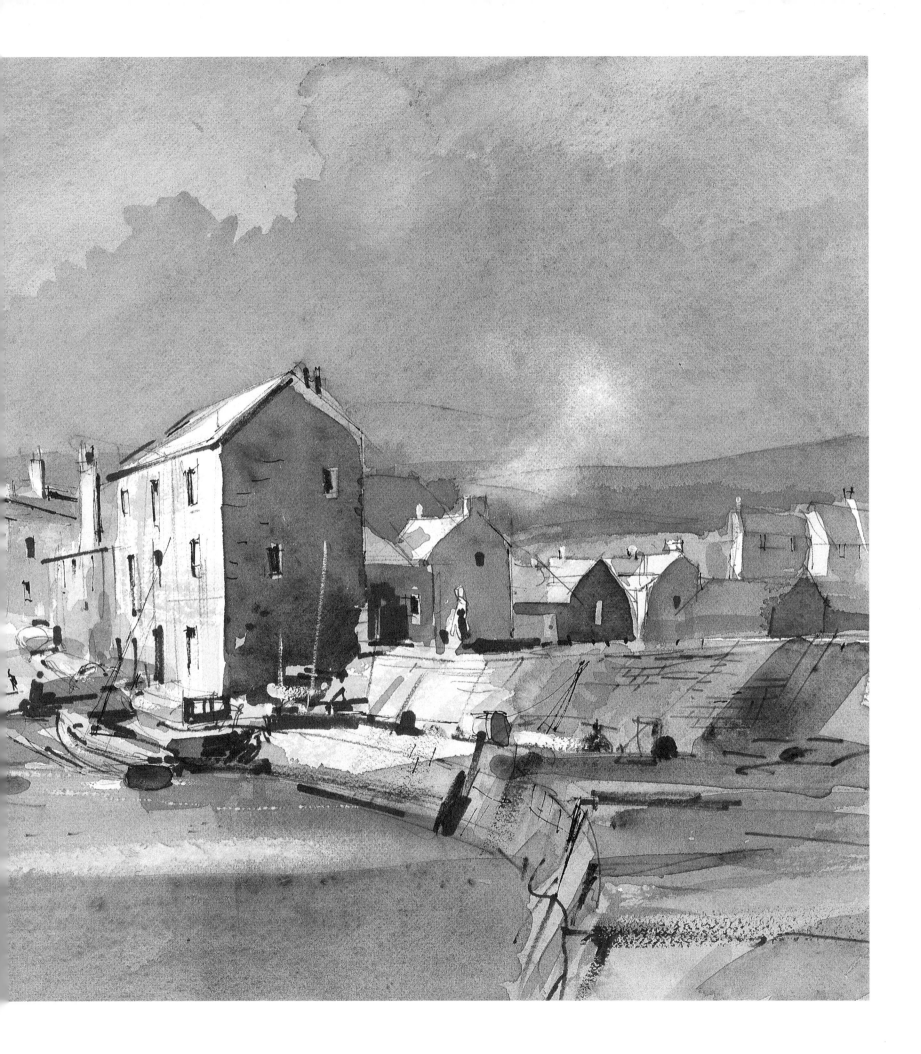

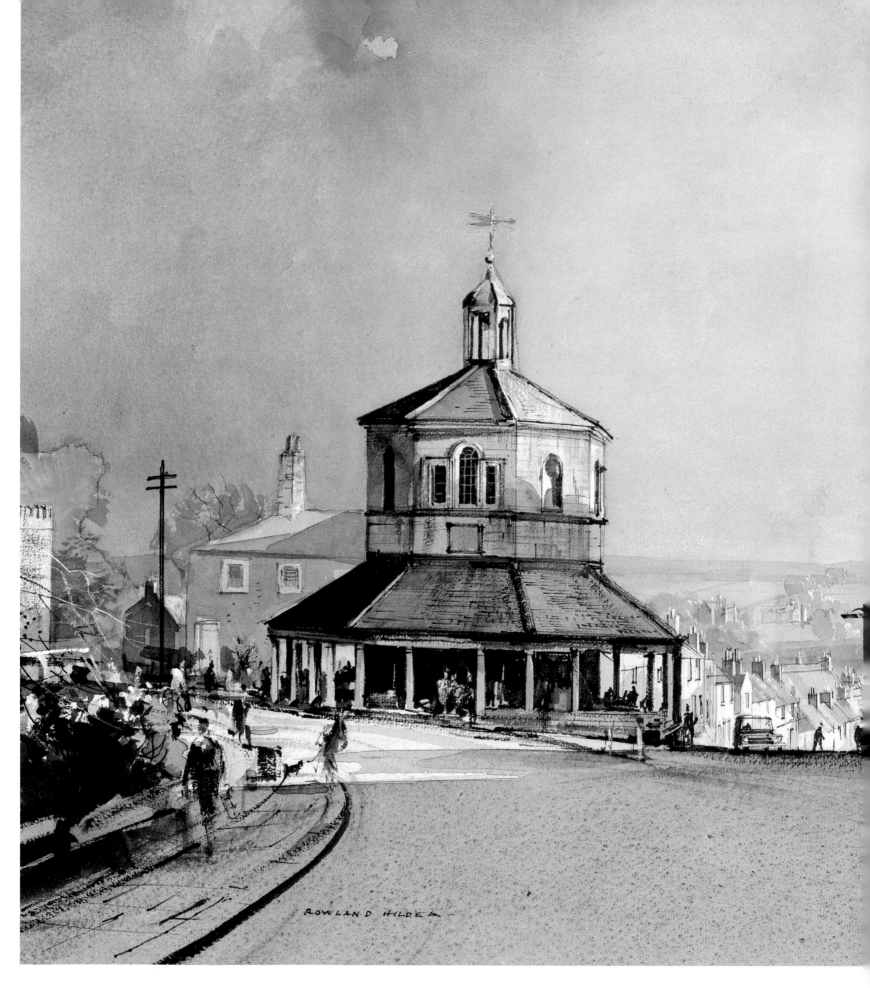

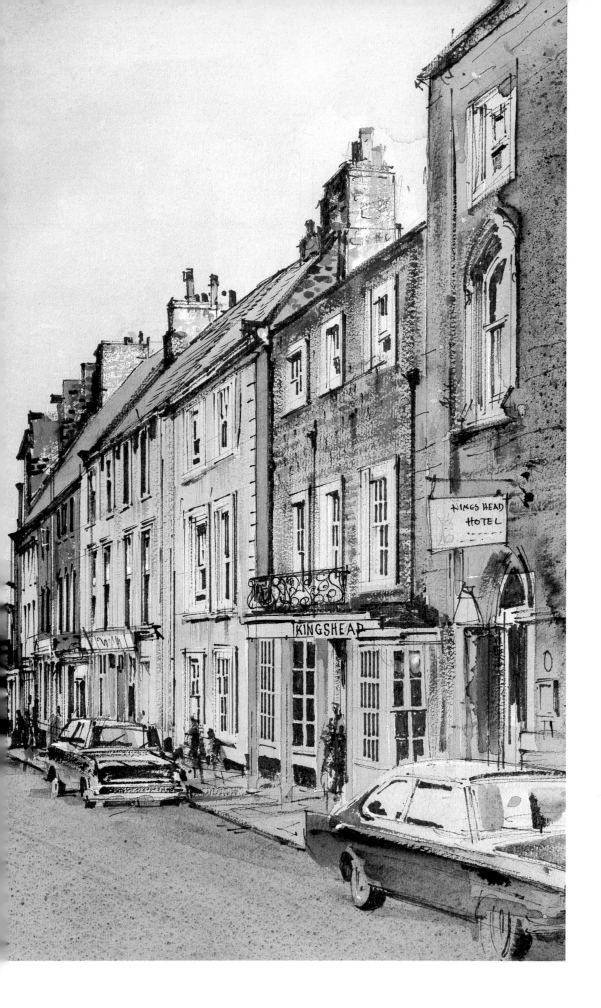

BARNARD CASTLE, DURHAM

There was a castle here before the town, but little of it remains except bits of the great hall and a twelfth-century keep. Dickens researched *Nicholas Nickleby* here, including visits to the local boarding schools, one of which, Bowes Academy, became the model for Dotheboys Hall and its proprietor the real-life original of the monstrous Mr Wackford Squeers.

THE GREYHOUND INN, CORFE, DORSET (*overleaf*)

The inn, below the ruins of Corfe Castle, was converted two and a half centuries ago from a group of cottages built in the 1650s. One of the castle's claims on history is the murder there of the eighteen-year-old King Edward by his stepmother, Elfrida, in 987. Wicked old King John later turned the place into a treasure store and torture chamber.

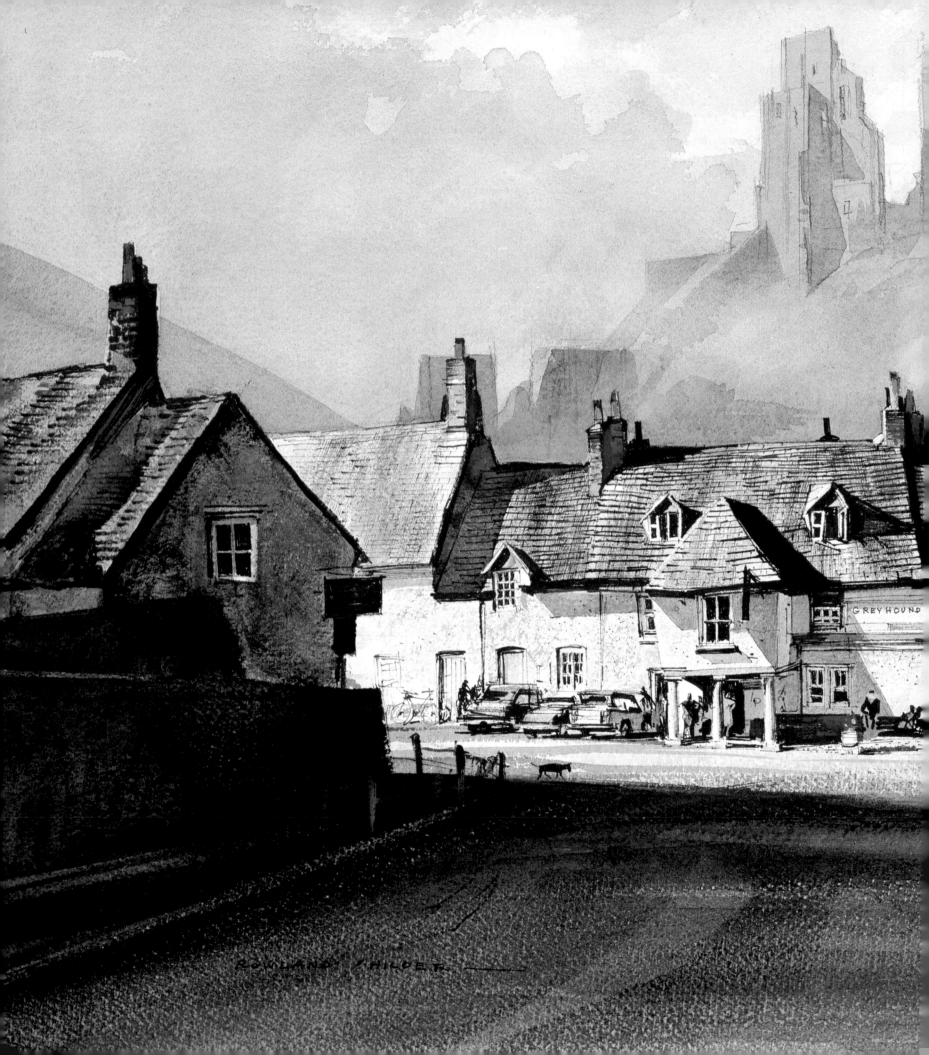

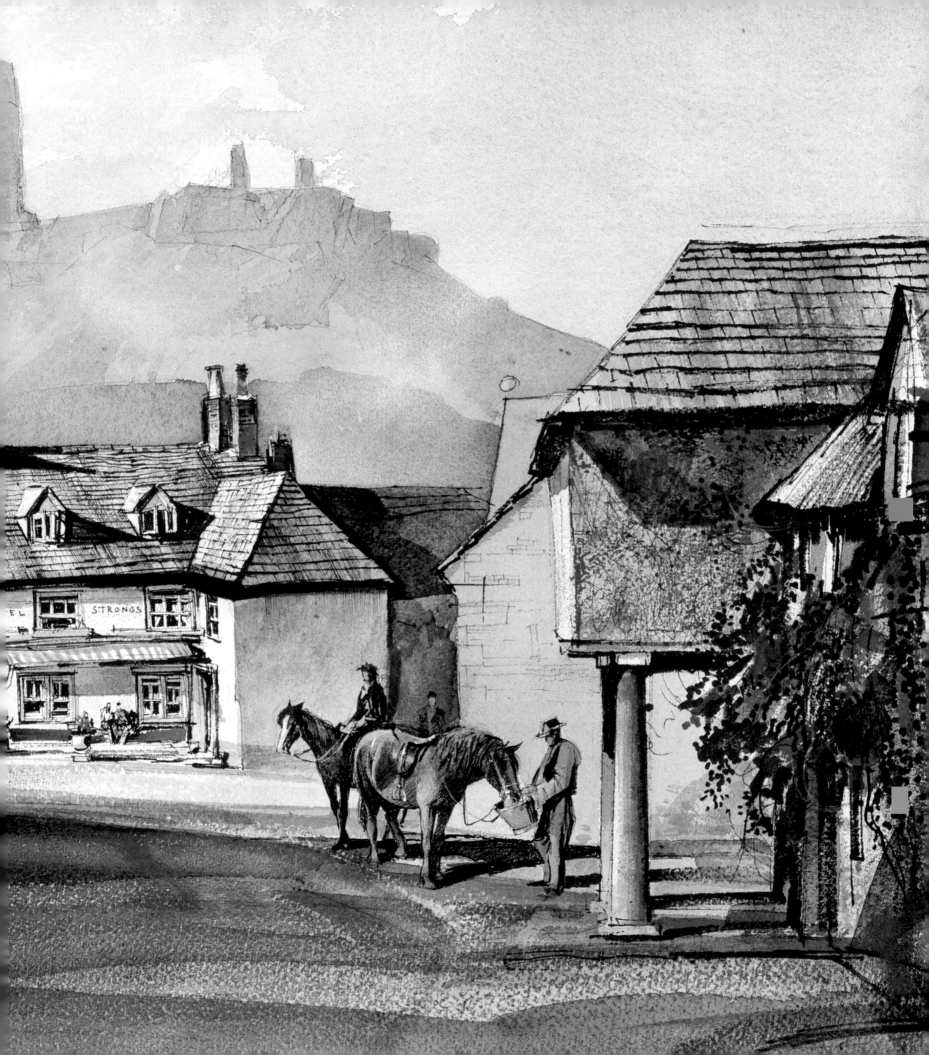

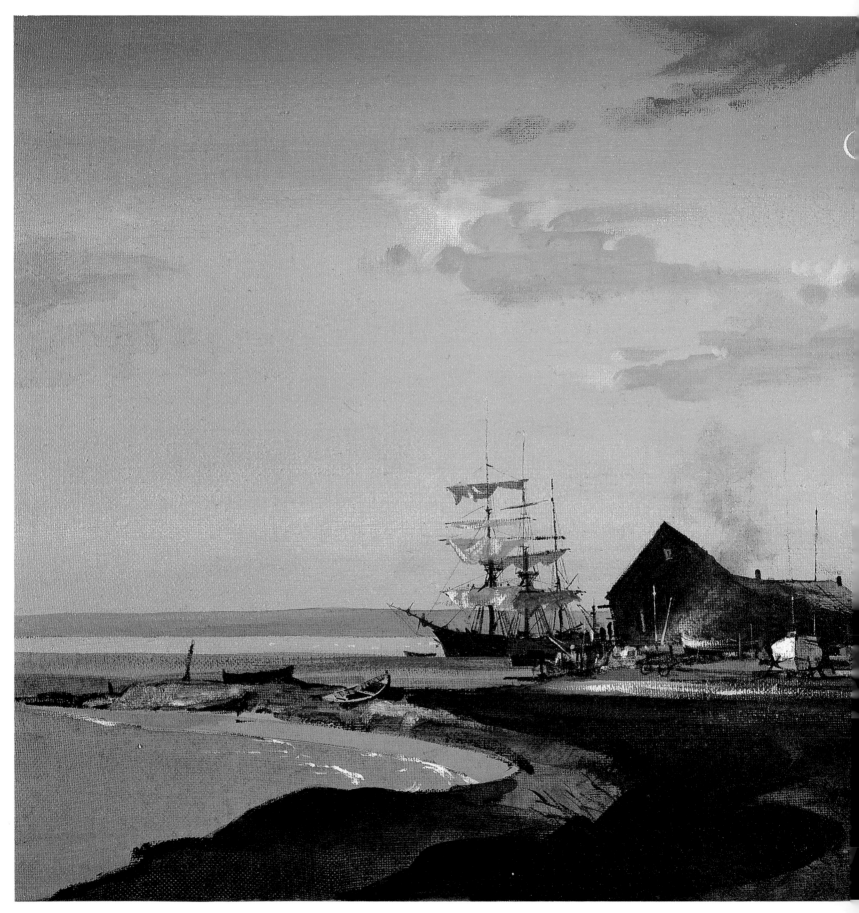

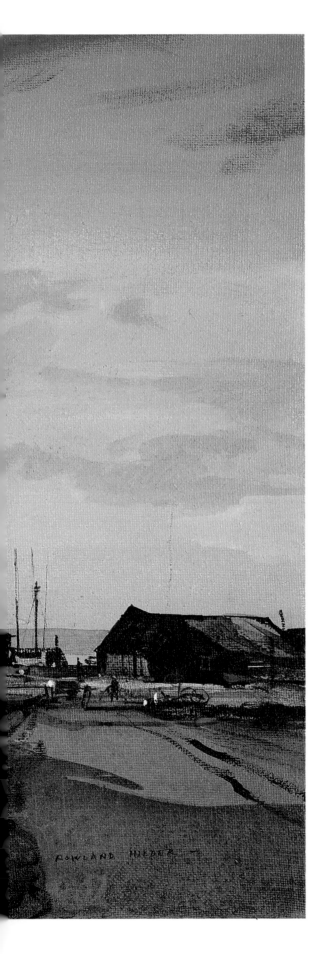

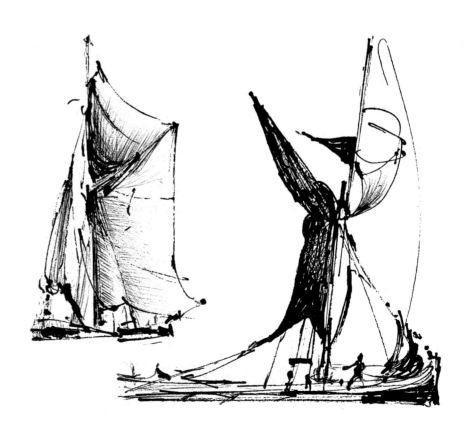

COBB'S QUAY

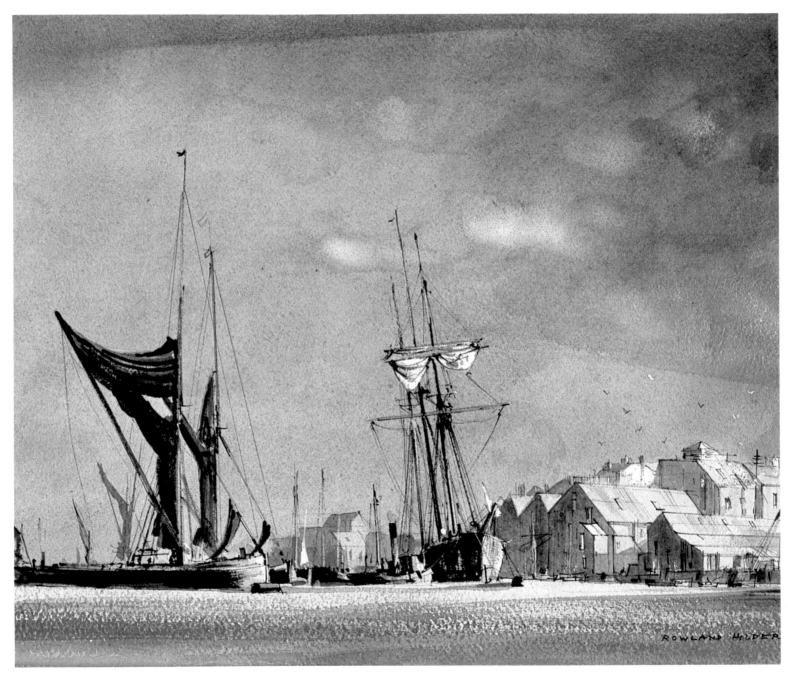

THE MEDWAY, 1928

BANKS AND BRAES

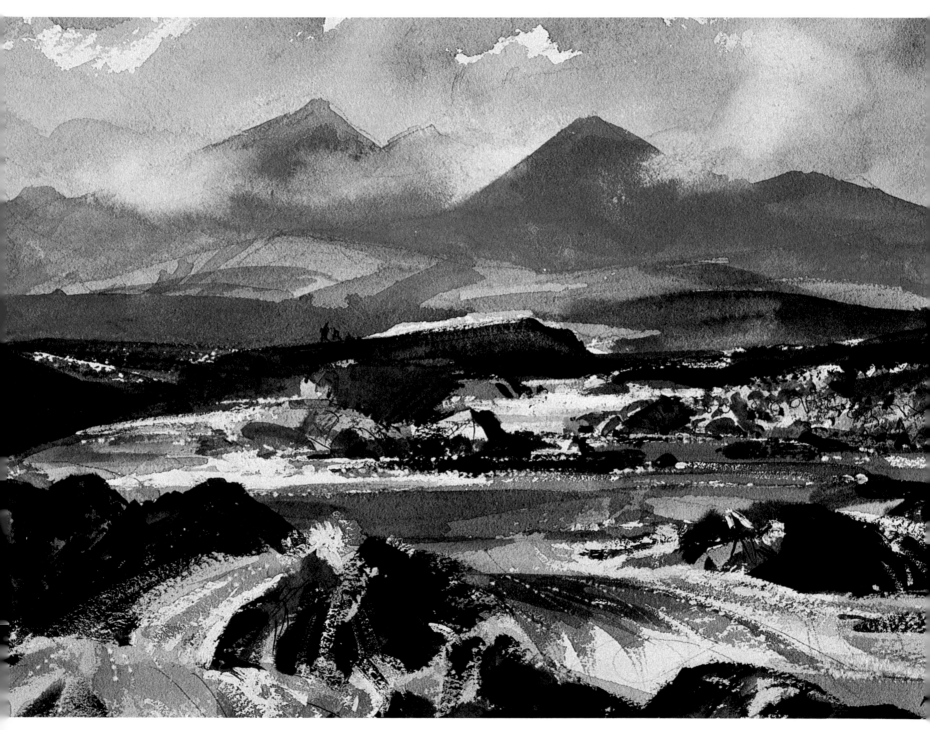

THE HIGHLANDS: RIVER IN SPATE

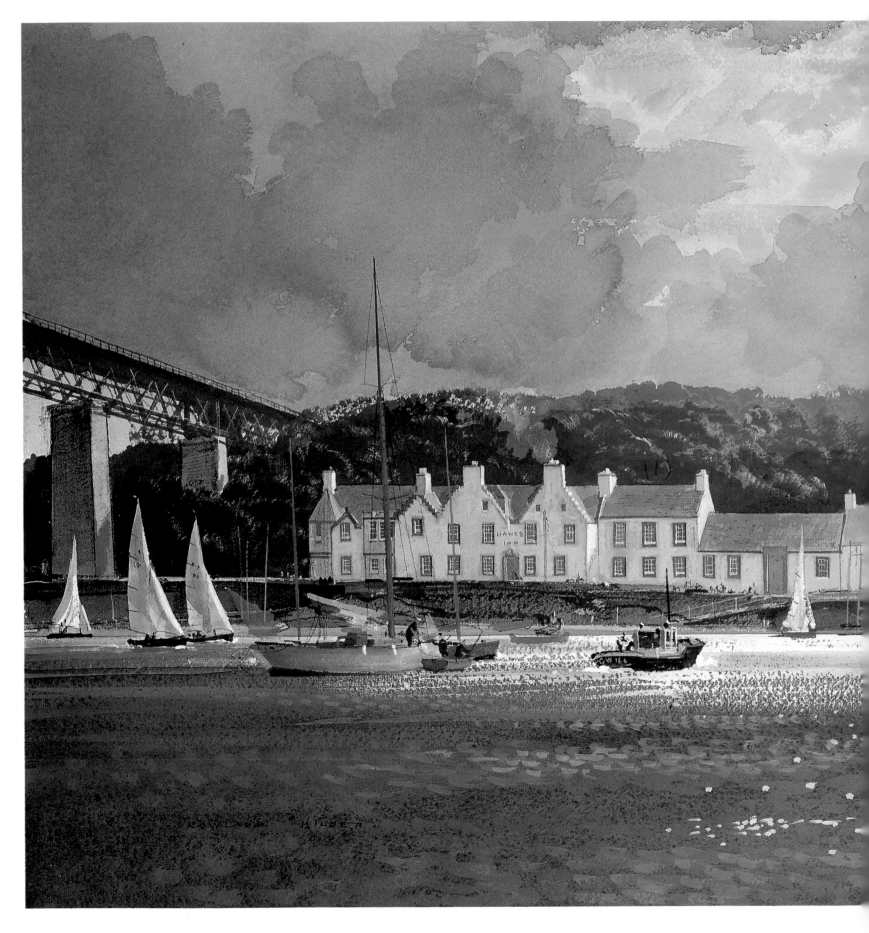

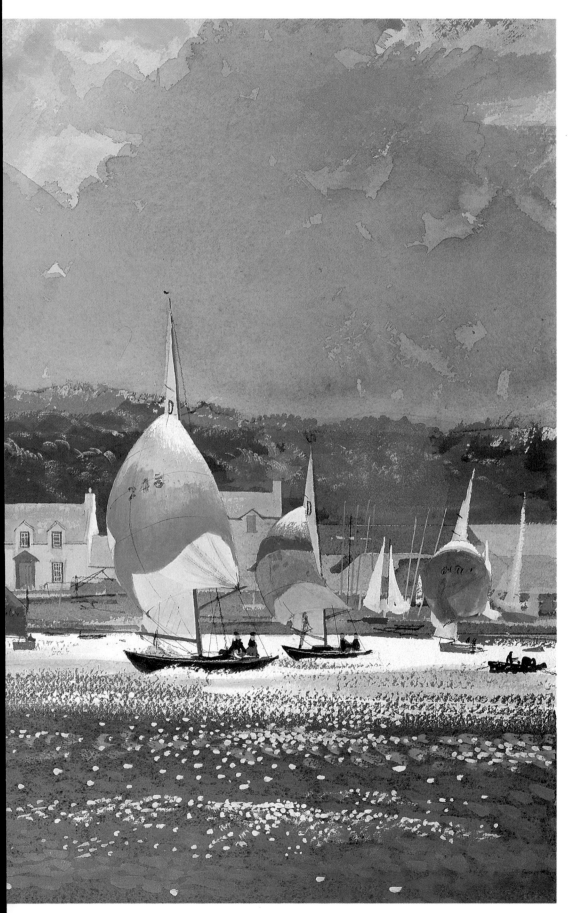

SOUTH QUEENSFERRY, WEST LOTHIAN: HAWES INN

Visitors of a literary mind can look up the pub in *Kidnapped*, chapter five. It is reputedly over three hundred years old, and occupies a position where the Firth of Forth narrows to the width of a river, turning the upper reach into a land-locked haven for anglers and yachtsmen.

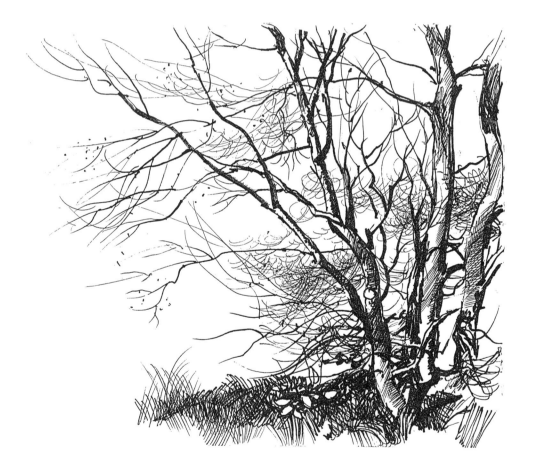

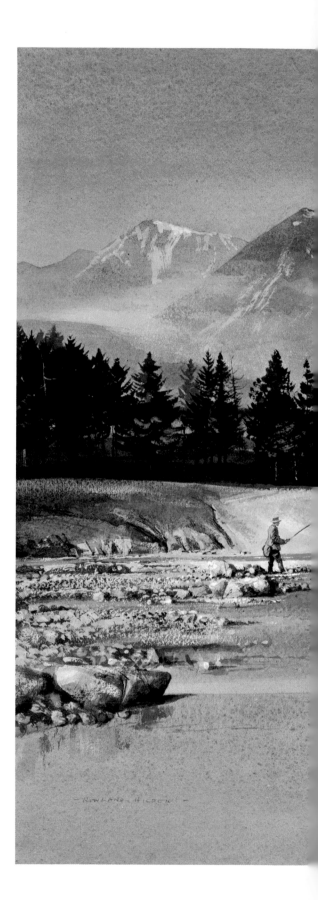

RANNOCH MOOR, PERTHSHIRE, AND THE KINGSHOUSE INN

It is a soggy place for walking, with nothing, according to a character in
Robert Louis Stevenson's *Kidnapped*, but 'heath, and crows, and Campbells'.

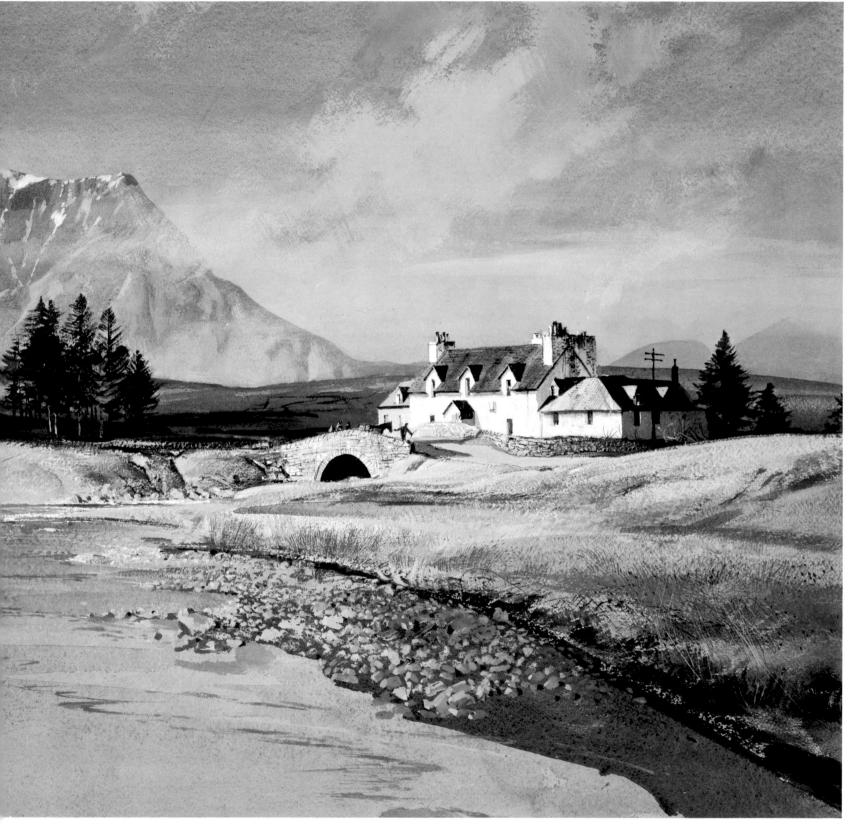

'What one draws is so often just a matter of where one happens to be, an individual response to a place one feels at home in.'

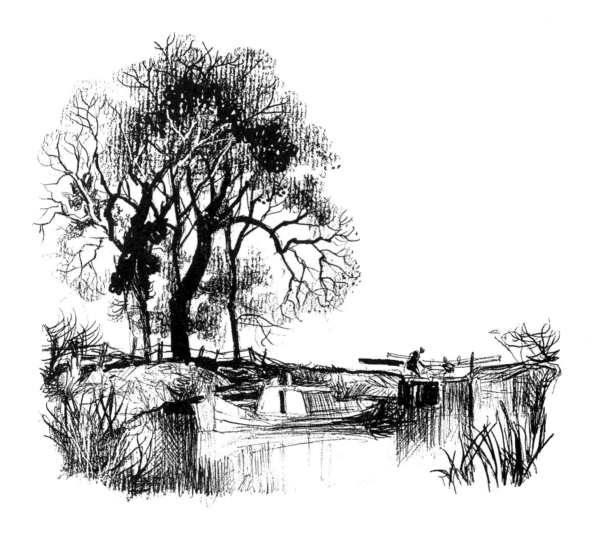

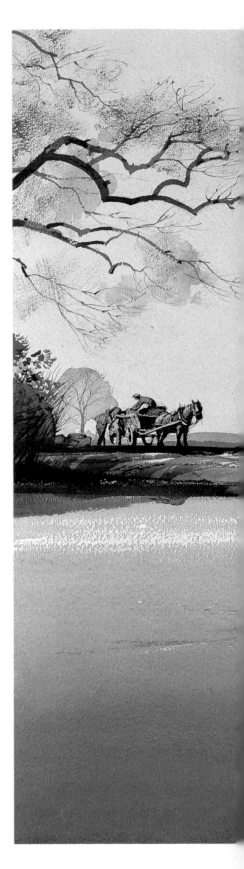

PRESTON MILL, EAST LINTON, LOTHIAN

This scene, looking rather as if it had been transported from the Weald of Kent, is of the sole surviving water-mill and barley kiln on the River Tyne, a favourite spot for artists, now in the care of the National Trust for Scotland.

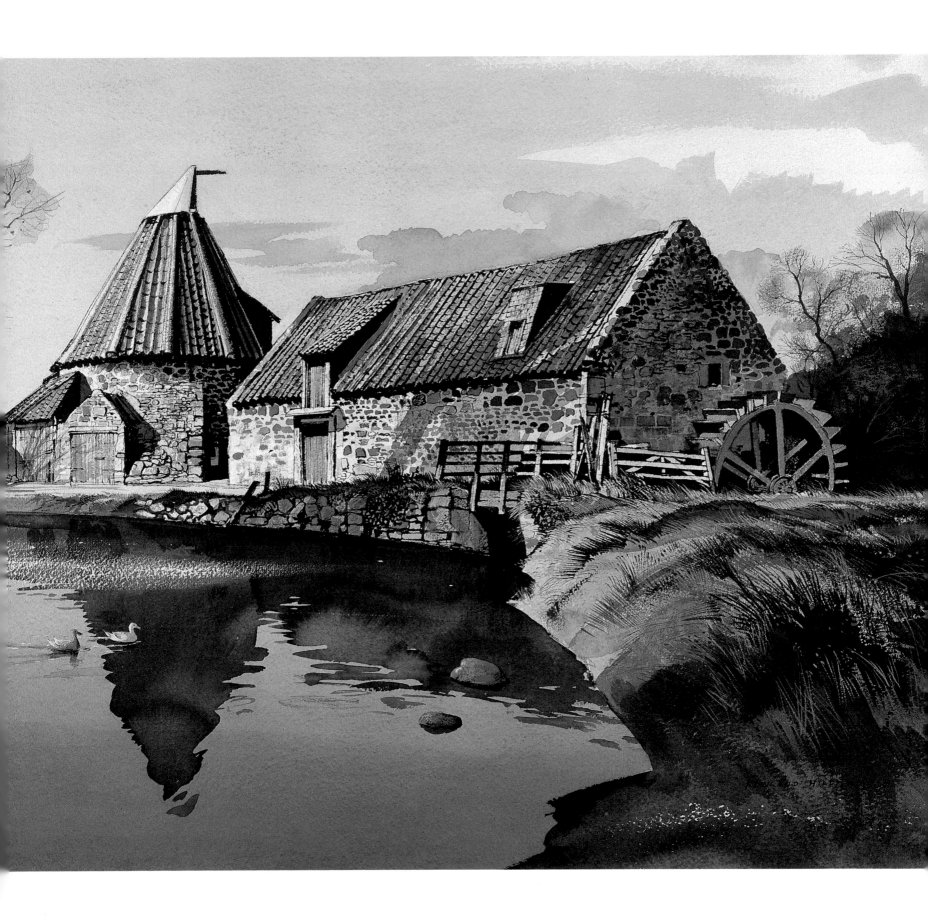

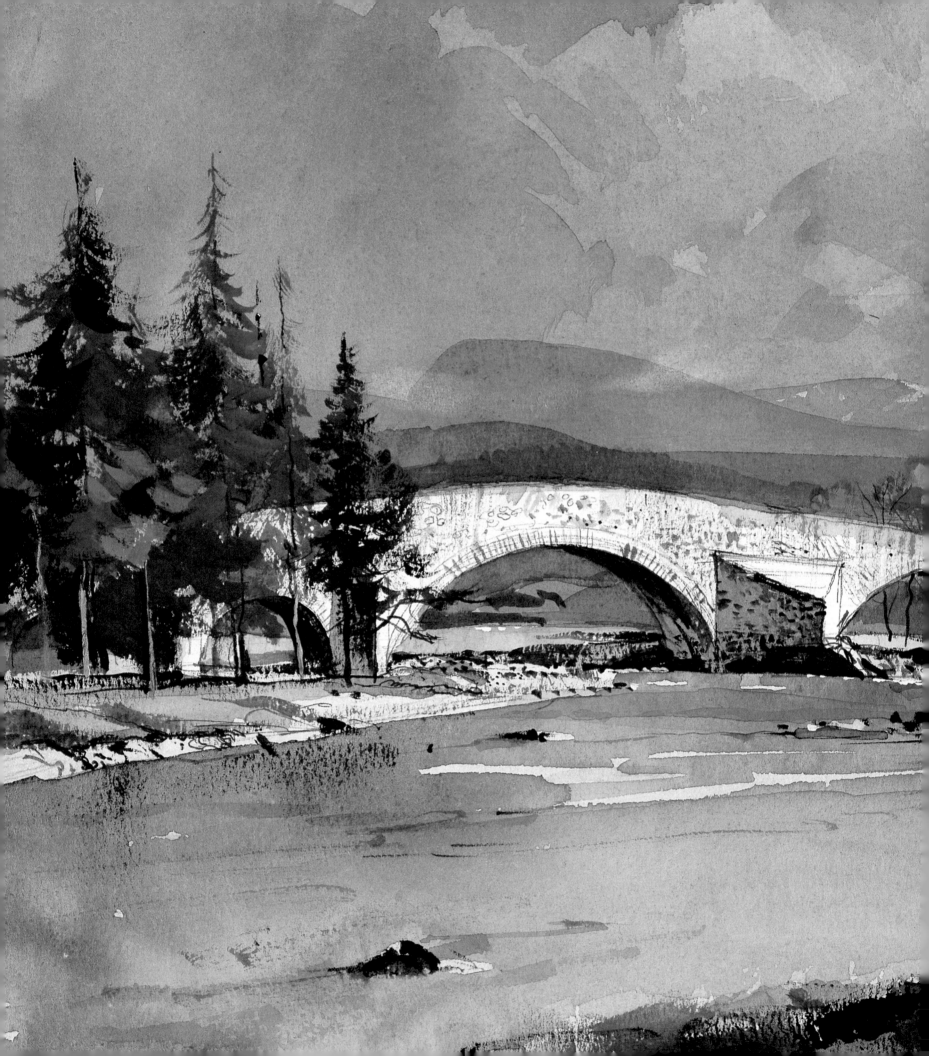

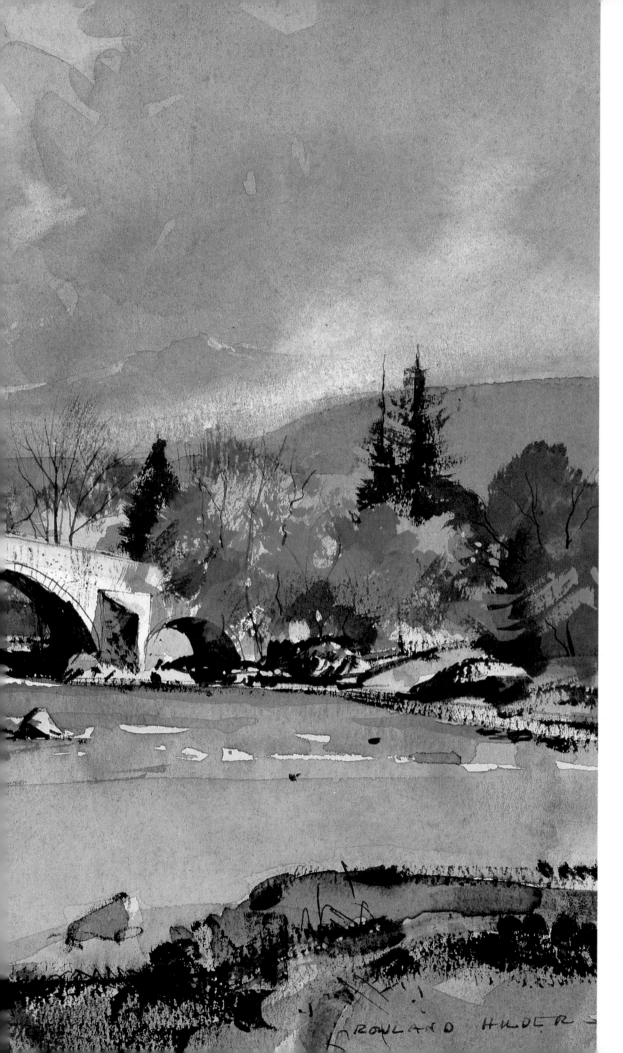

THE BRIG O'DEE
NEAR BRAEMAR

71

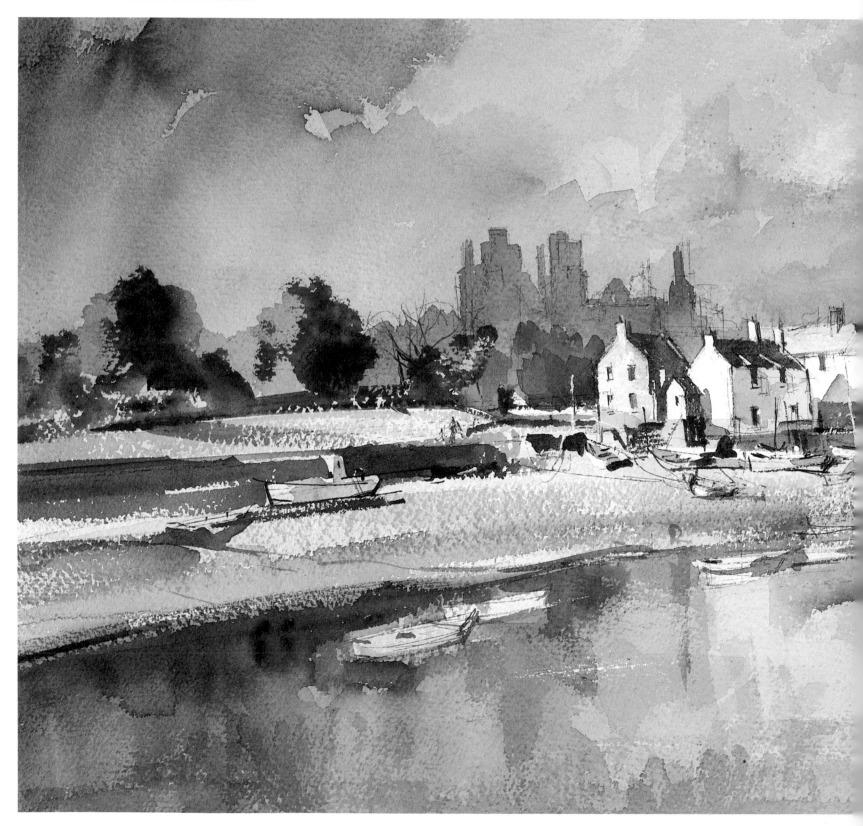

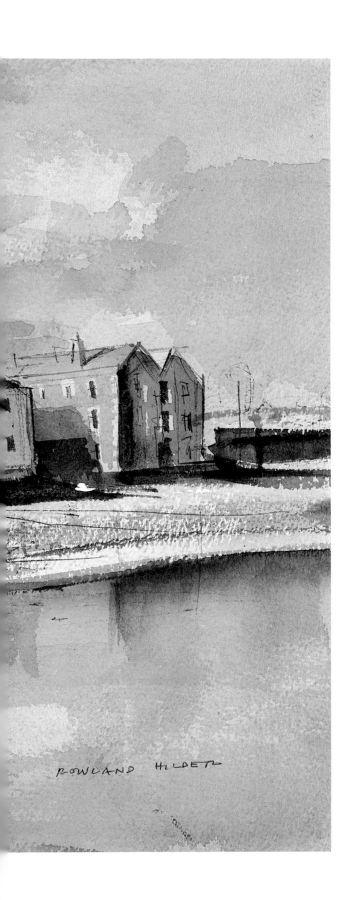

ROWLAND HILDER

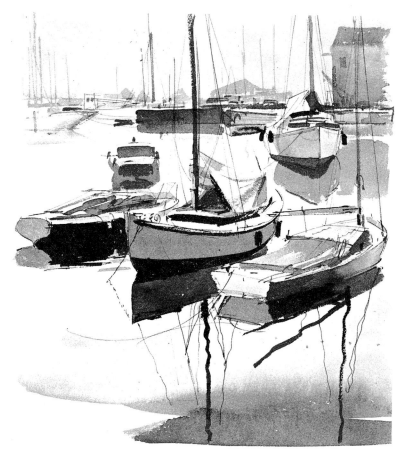

73

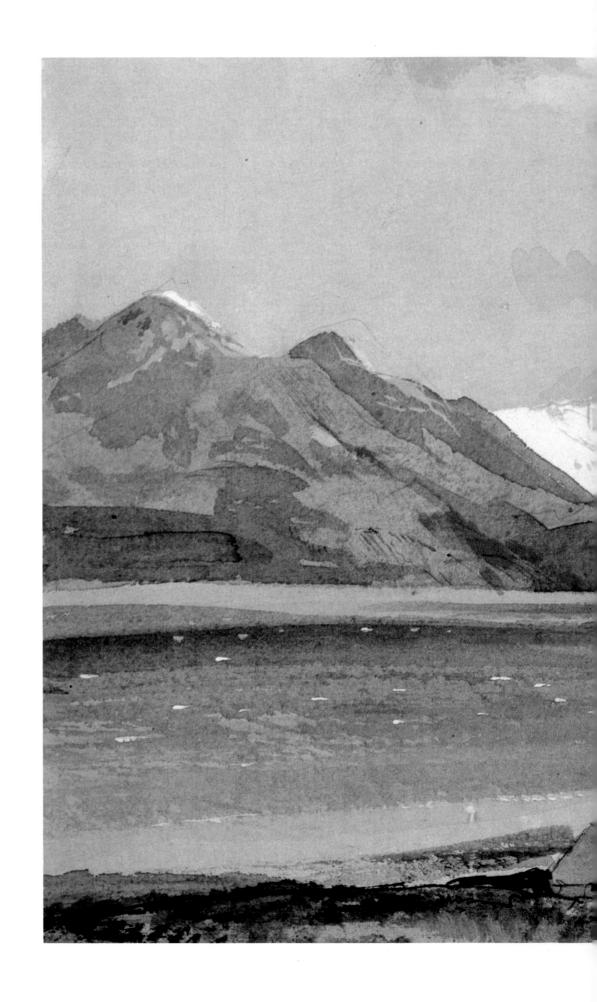

THE CUILLINS FROM LOCH
SCAVAIG, ISLE OF SKYE

74

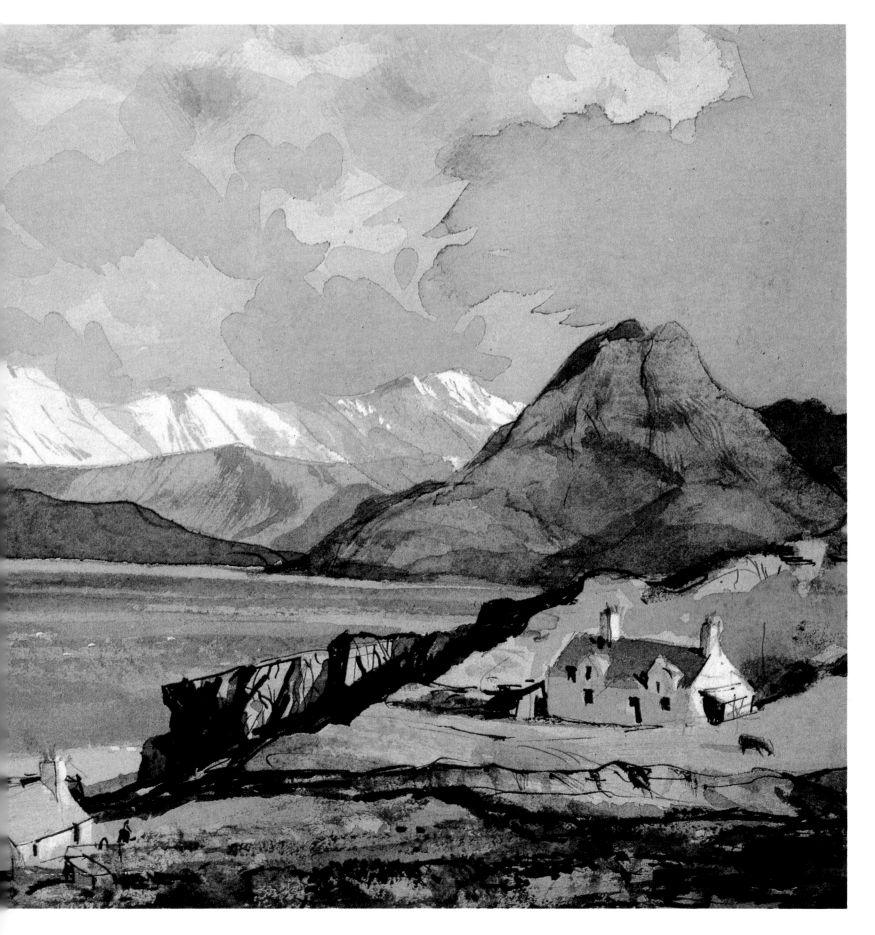

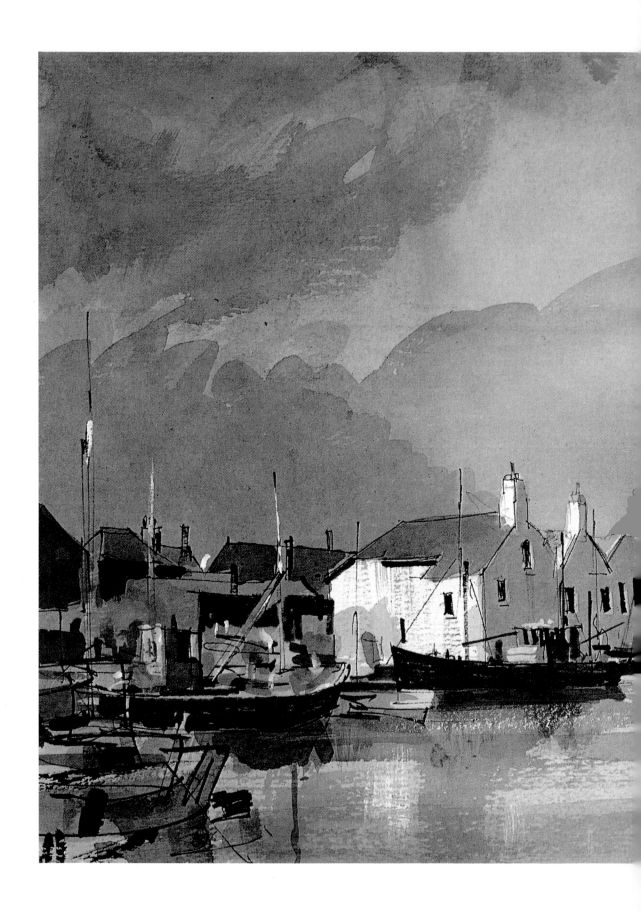

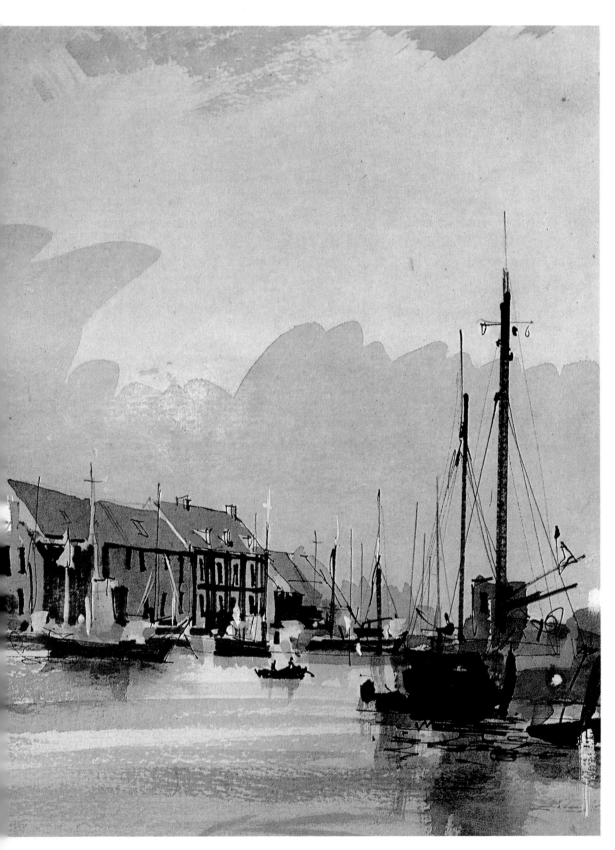

EYEMOUTH, BERWICKSHIRE

Sadness still seems to hang over the little fishing town. On October 14th 1881, twelve of its twenty-four fishing vessels were overwhelmed by a storm, with the loss of a hundred and twenty-nine men. It also has a well-merited reputation for smuggling.

STIRLING BRIDGE

This was the scene of one of those far-off battles against their southern neighbours that Scotsmen never forget. In 1297 Sir William Wallace overcame an English army under the command of the Earl of Surrey, softening up the Sassenachs for the battle of Bannockburn seventeen years later.

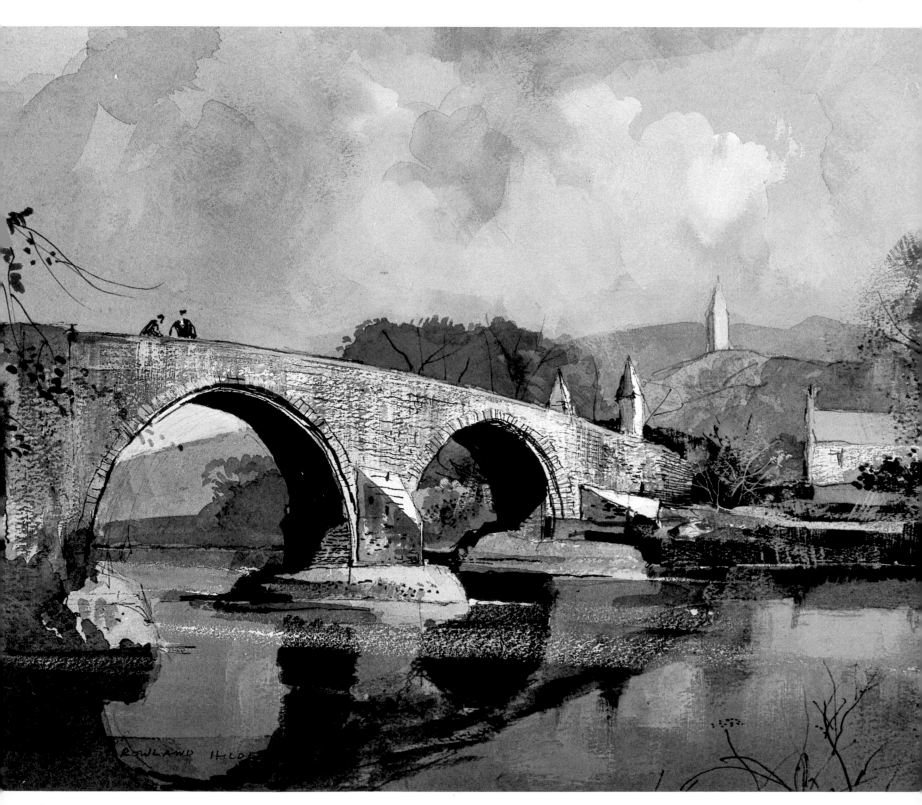

FOUR SEASONS

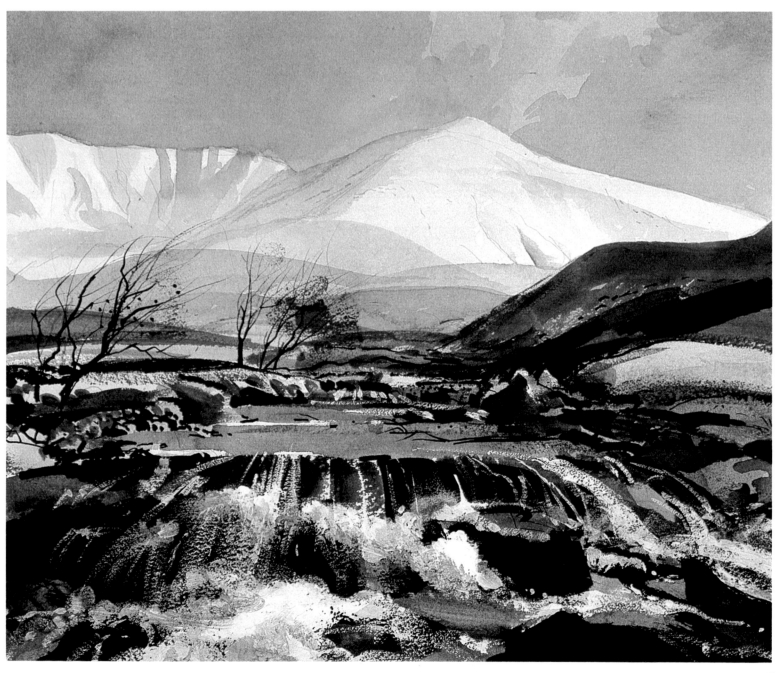

SONGS OF SPRING

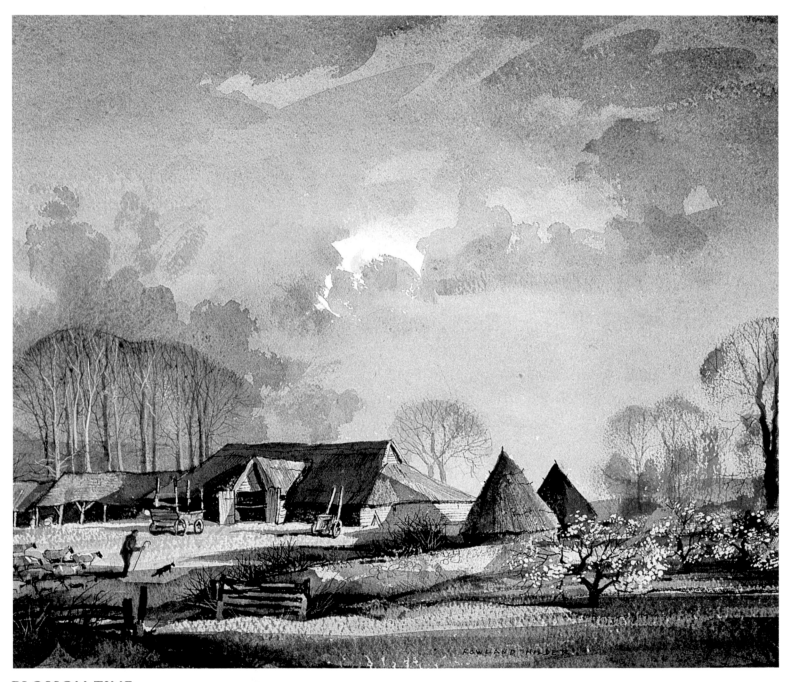

BLOSSOM TIME

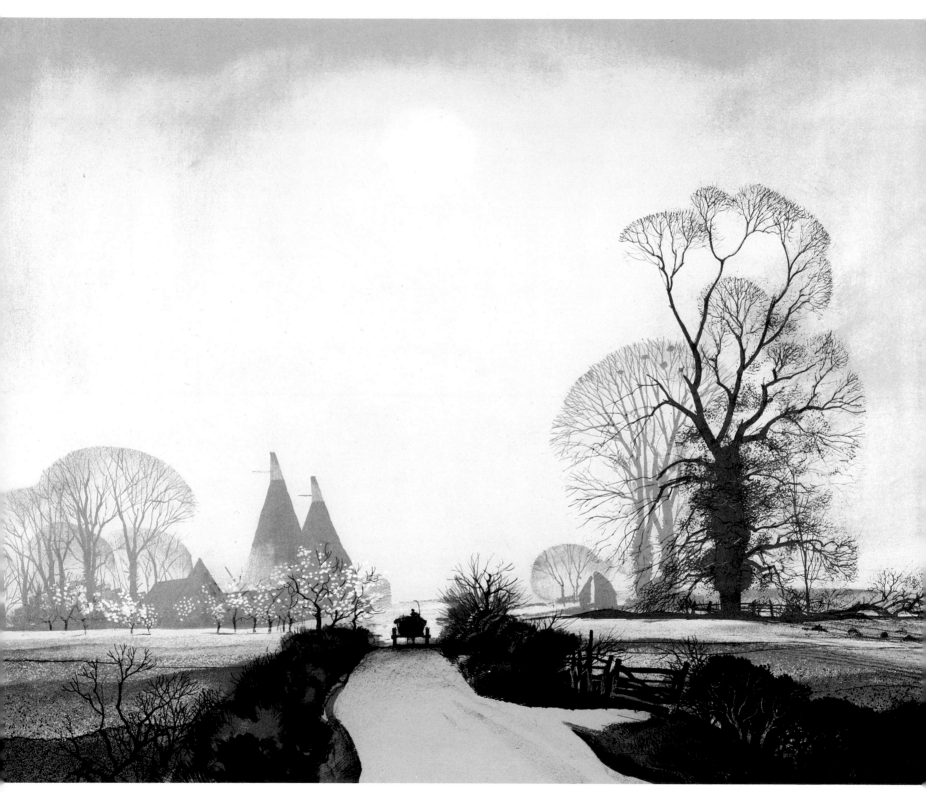

THE WEALD OF KENT

SUMMER ON THE ARUN

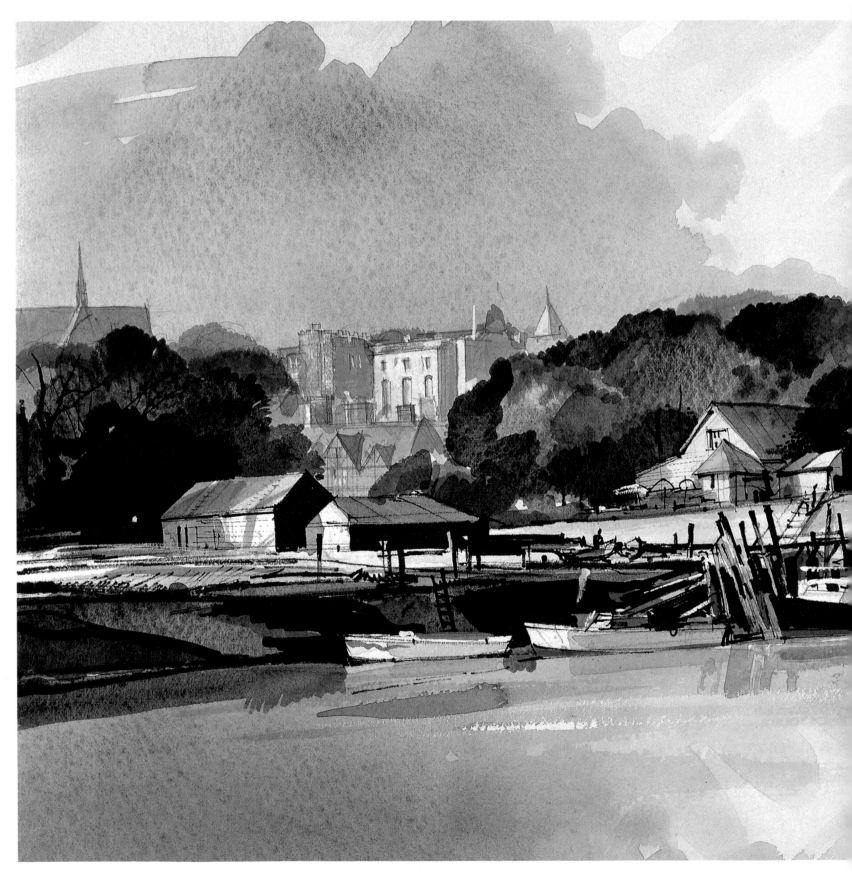

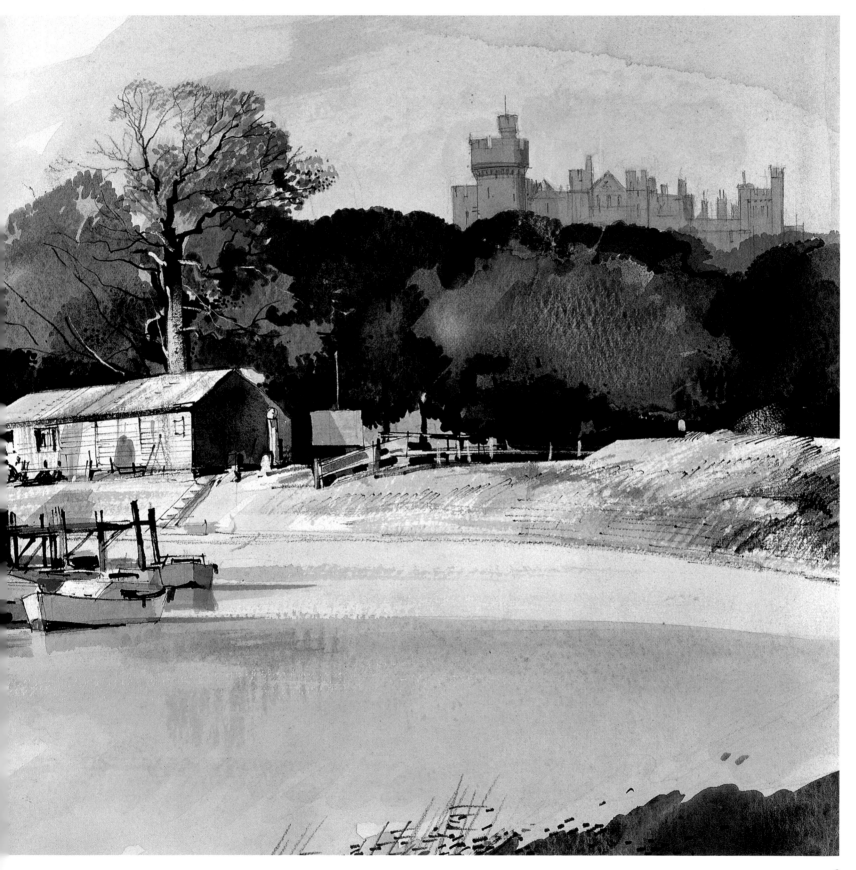

THE FALL OF THE YEAR

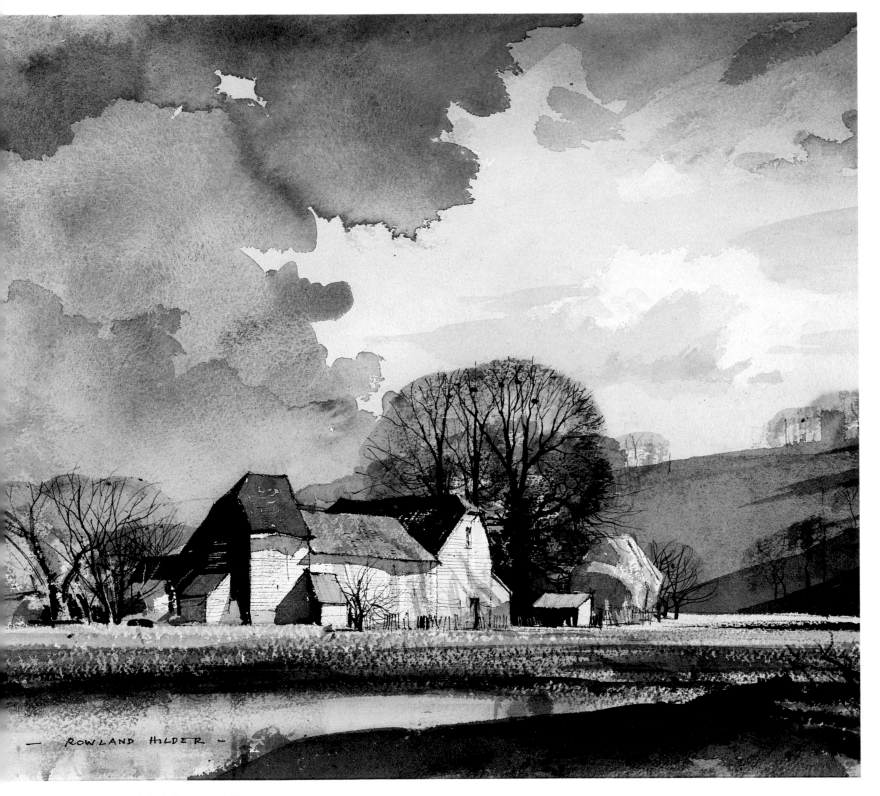

ROWLAND HILDER

BARNS IN AUTUMN

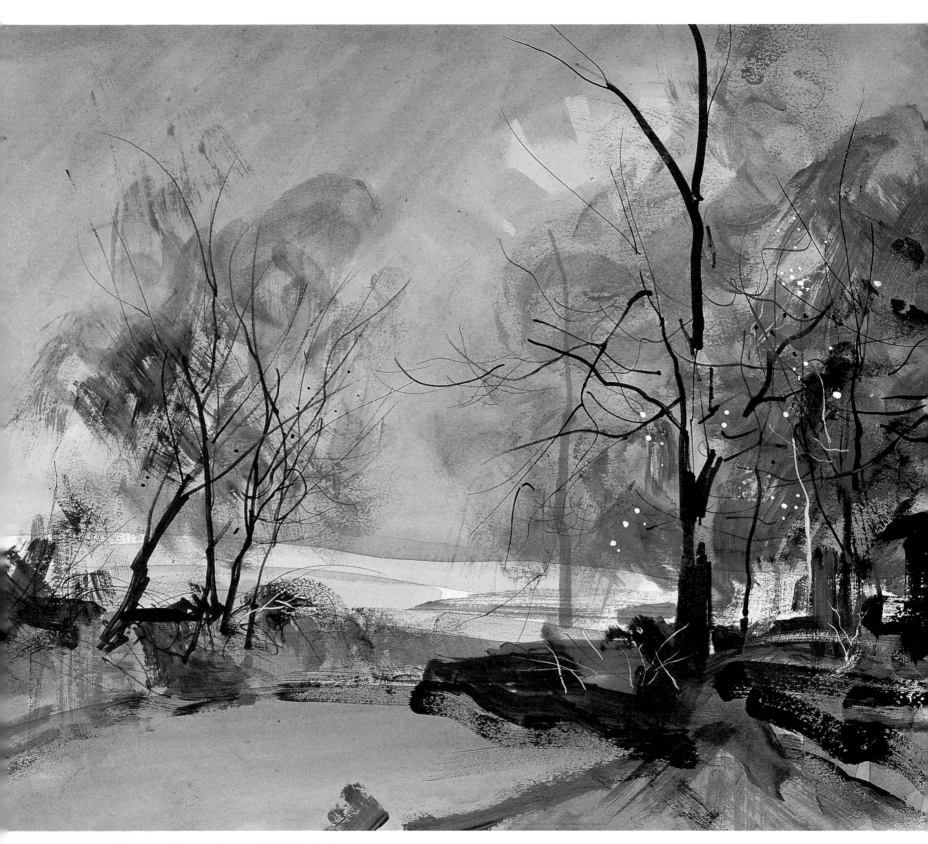

CULVERDOWN, NEAR SUDBURY

HARMONIES OF WINTER

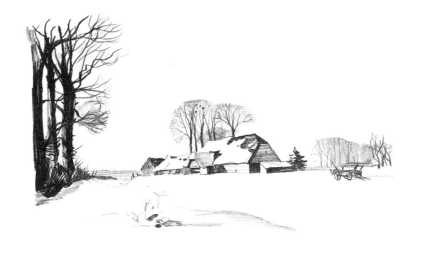

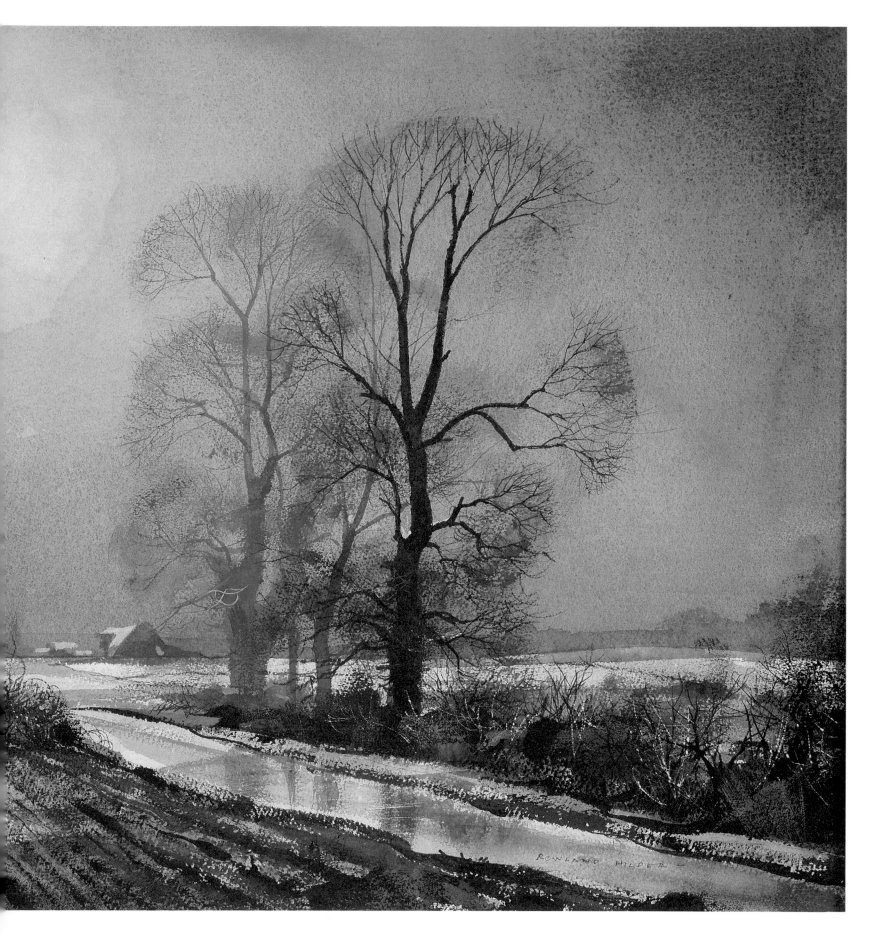

'The English winter opened my eyes
to a subject that, so far as I could see,
no English artist had tackled before.'

OASTS UNDER SNOW
(*Overleaf*) LANE AT WESTERHAM

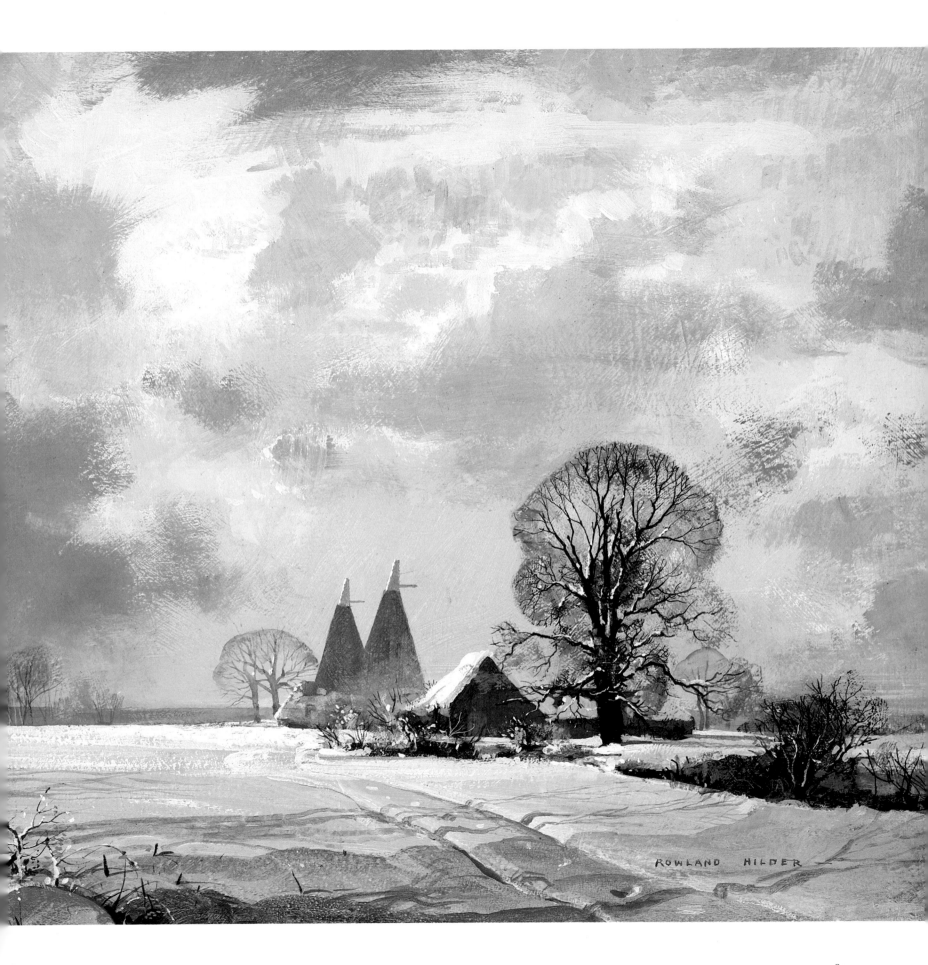

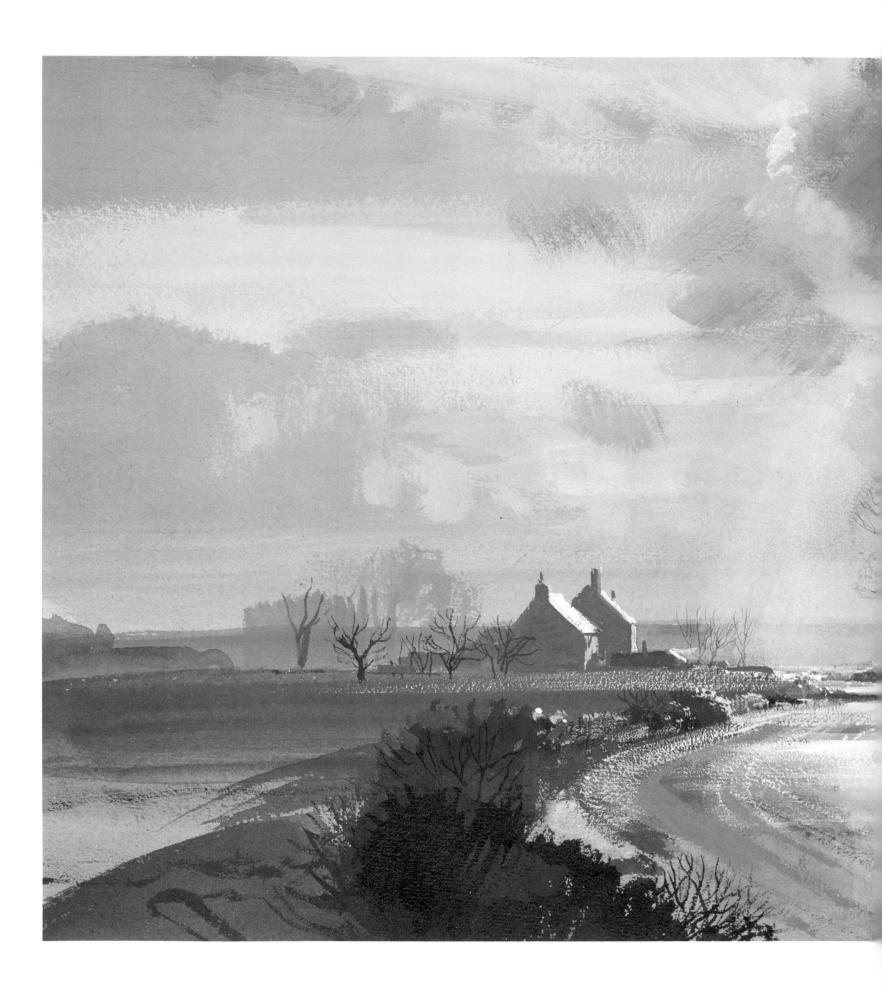

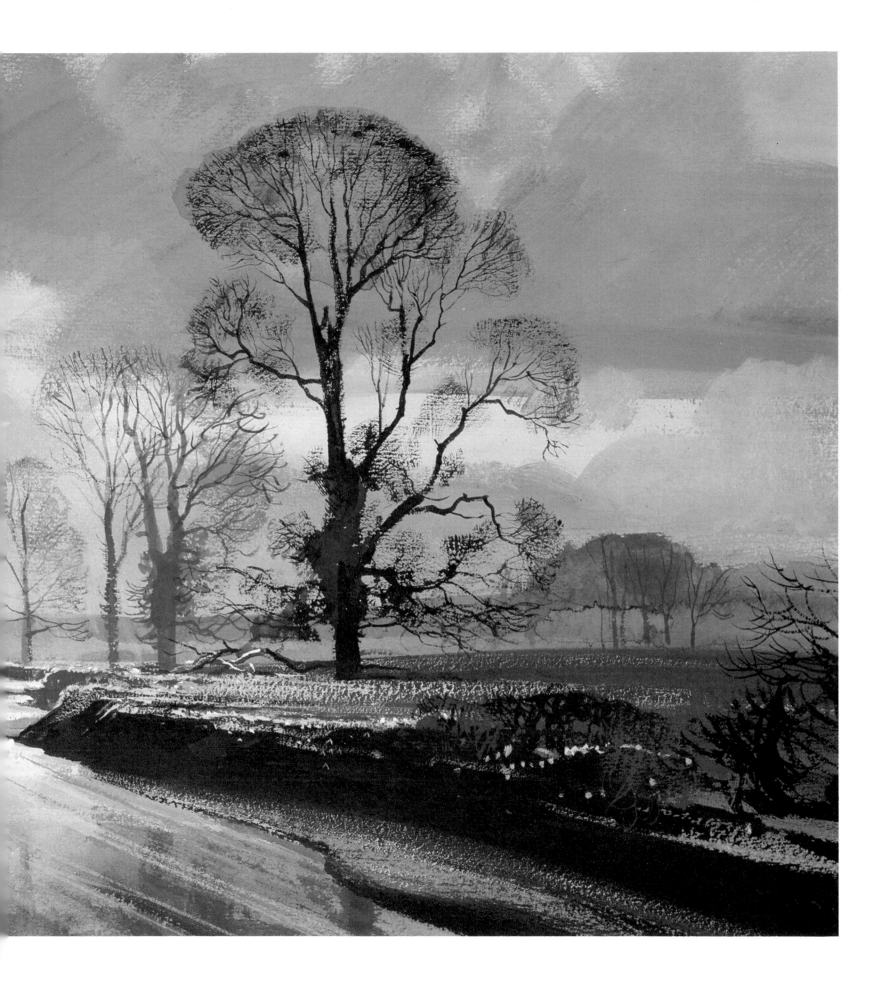

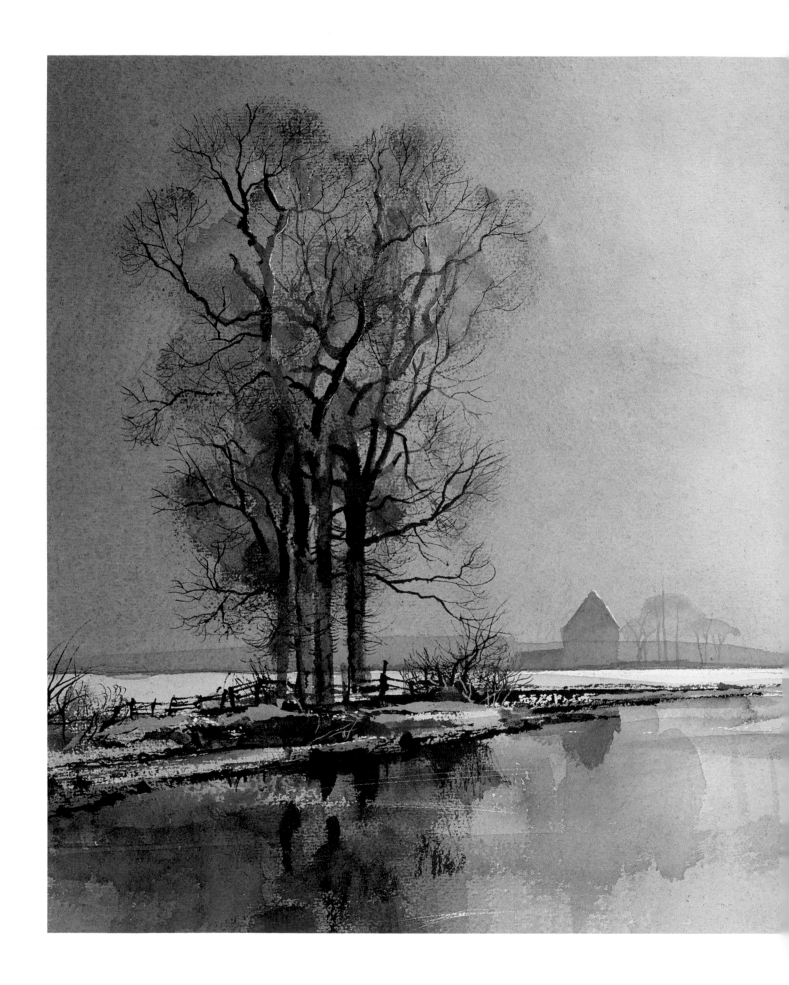

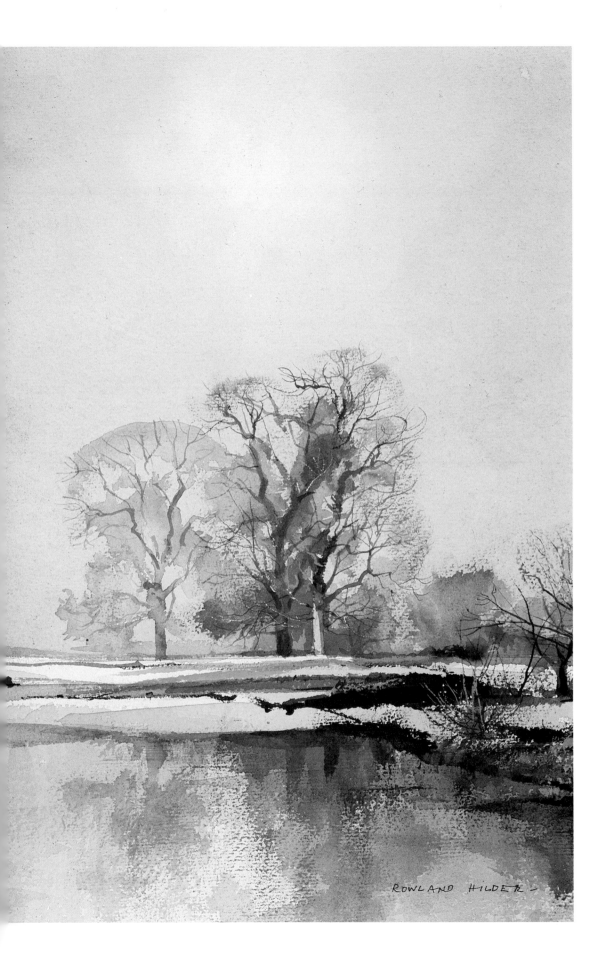

WINTER FLOOD

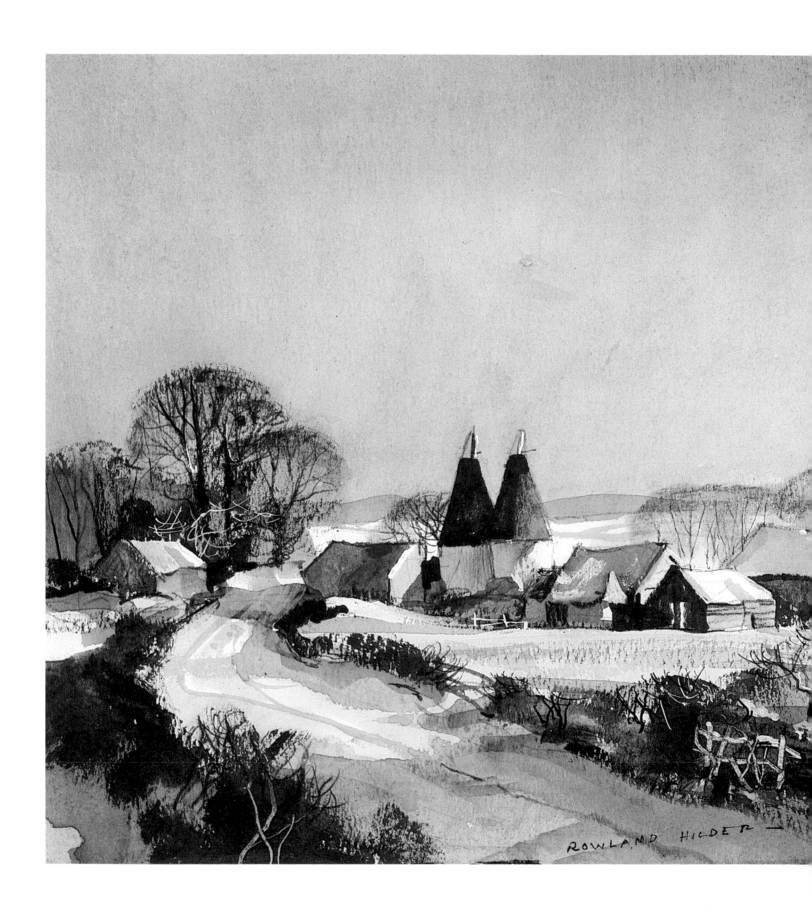

94

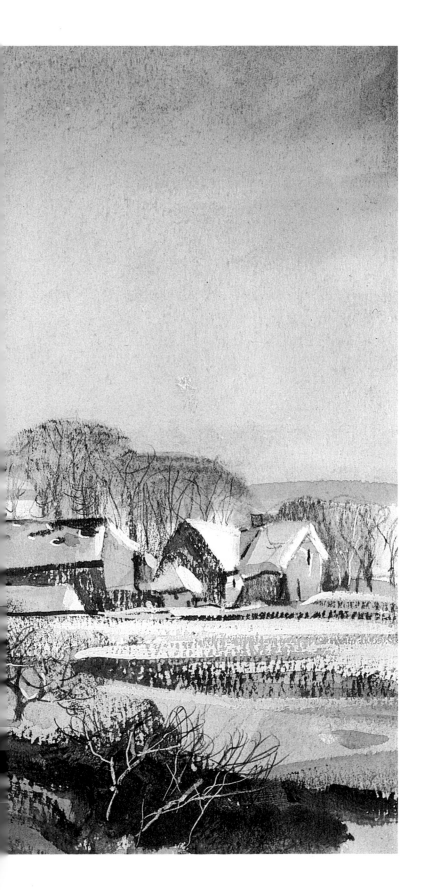

'The English countryside as I most
admired it, in its winter garb ...'

SNOW IN THE GARDEN OF ENGLAND

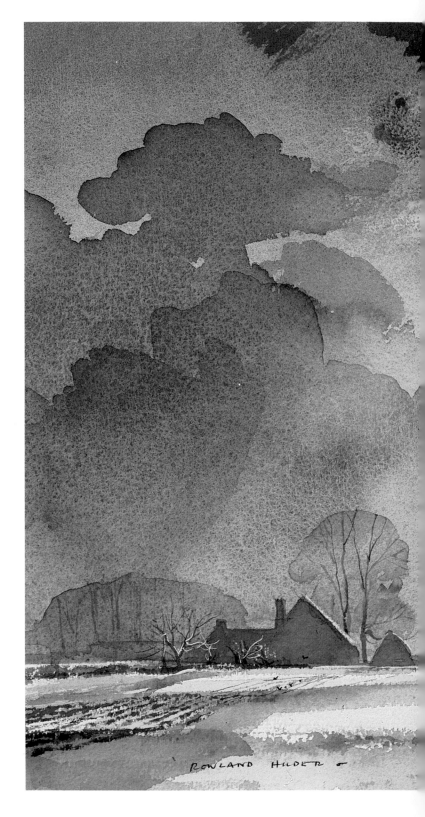

WINTER LANDSCAPE

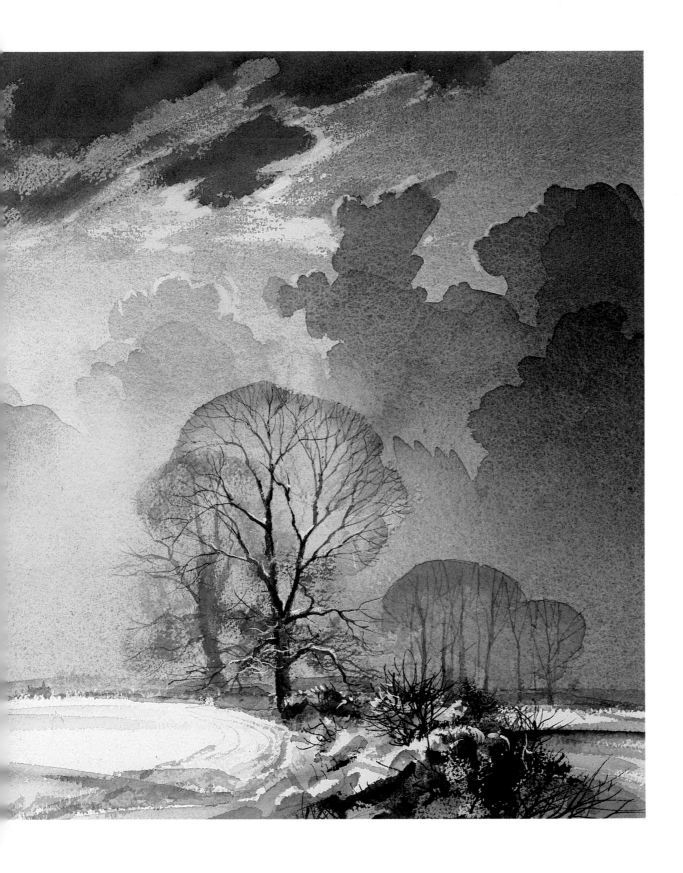

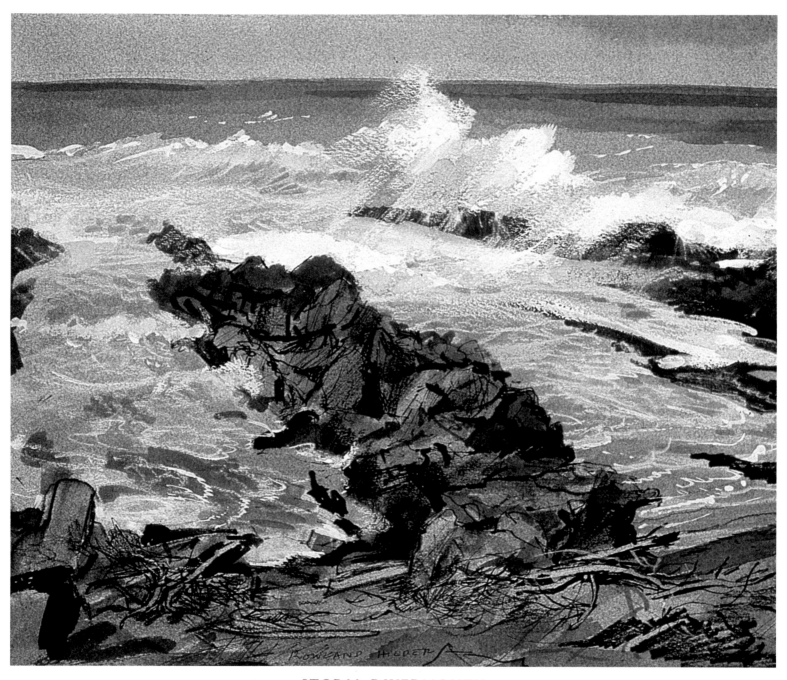

STORM, RIVERMOUTH

QUIET WATERS

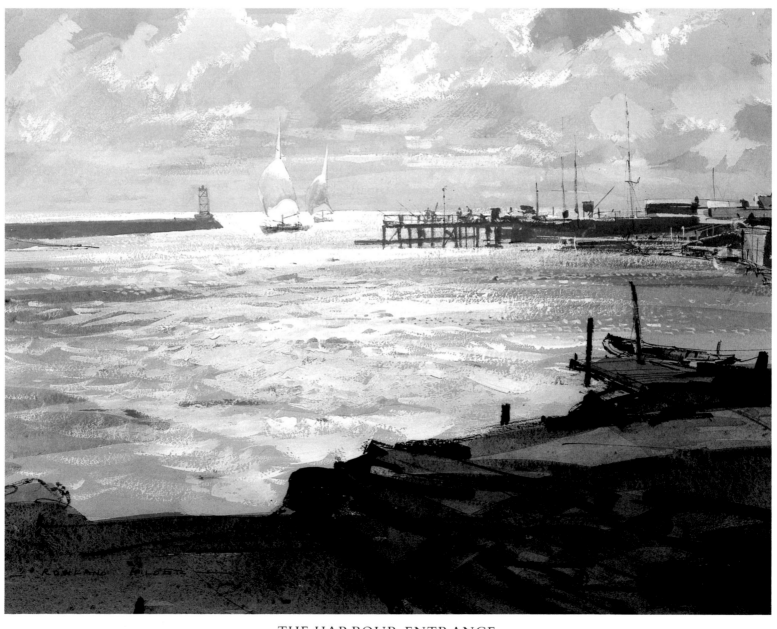

THE HARBOUR ENTRANCE

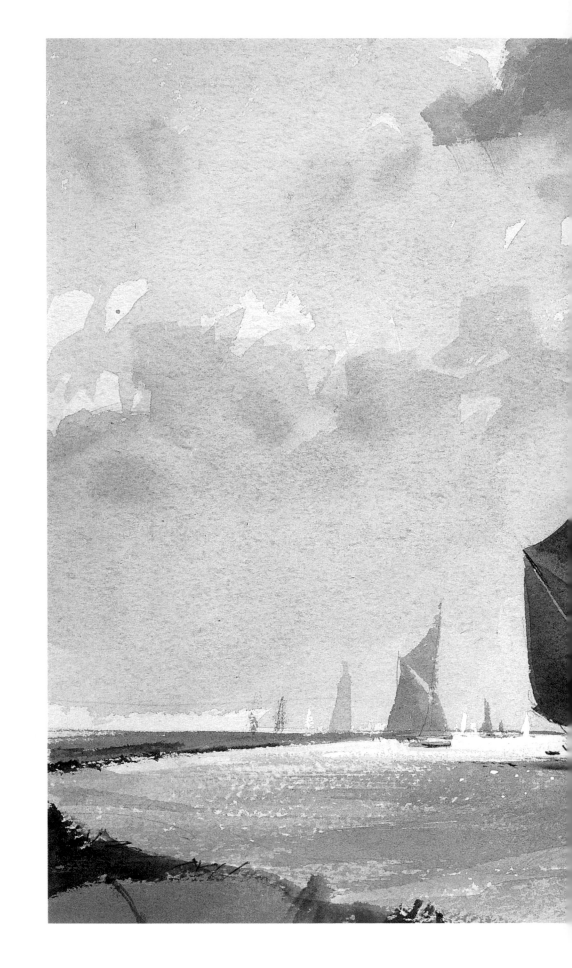

THE ESTUARY

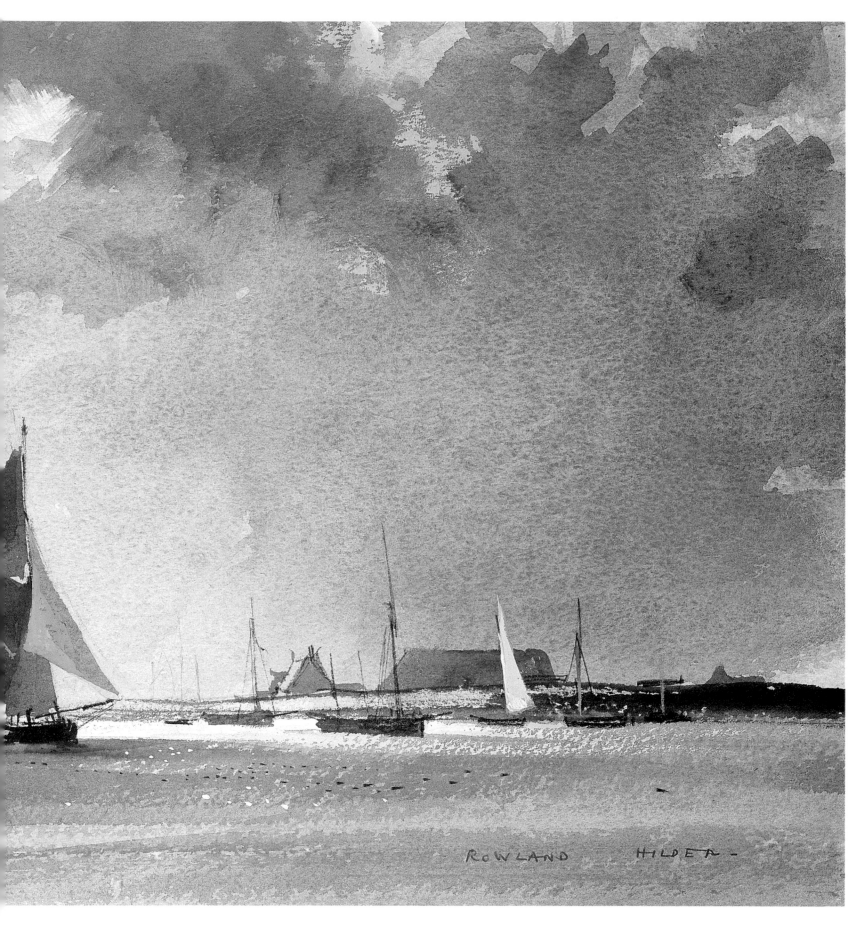

ROWLAND HILDER

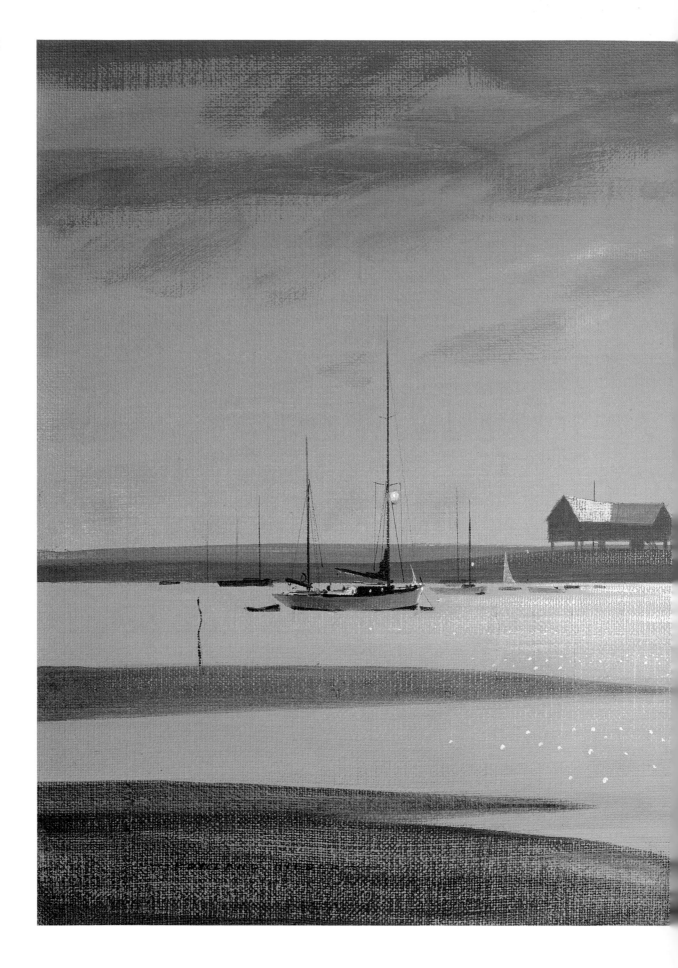

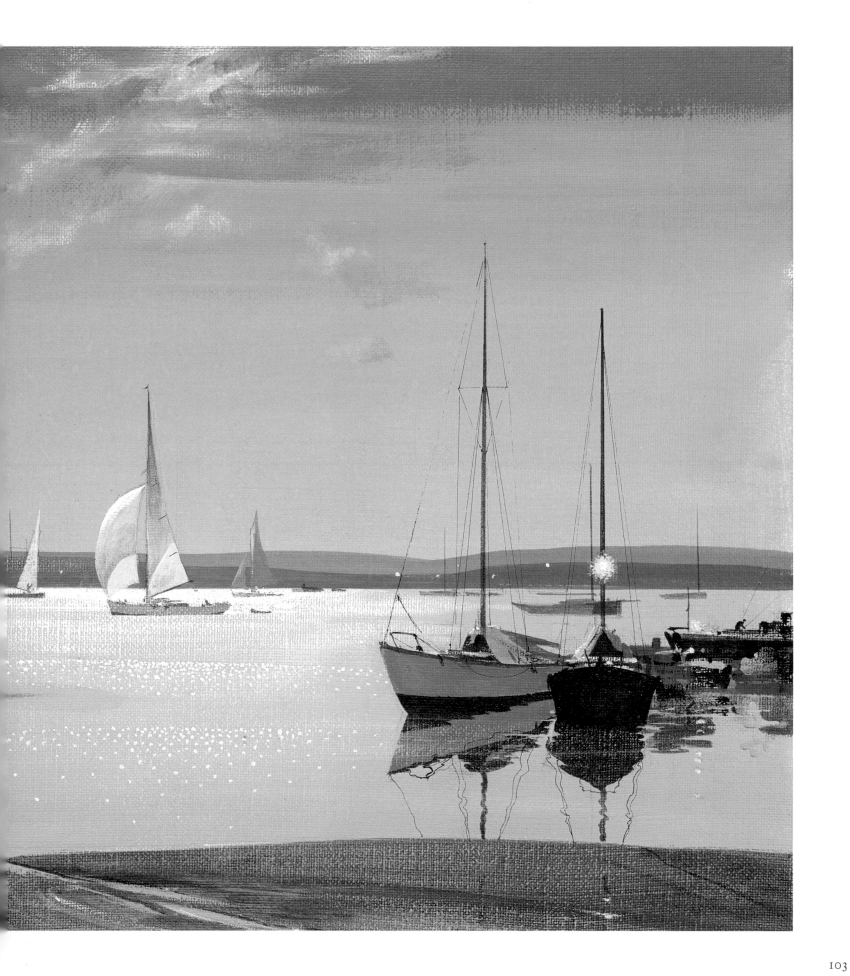

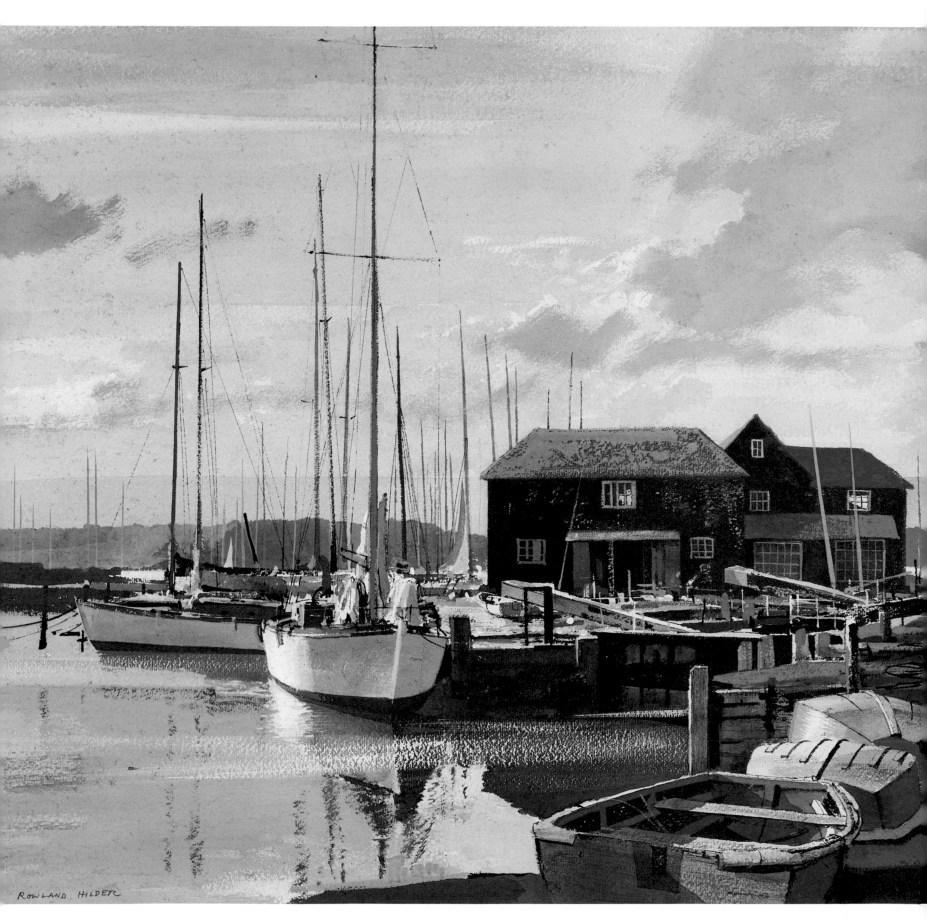

ROWLAND HILDER

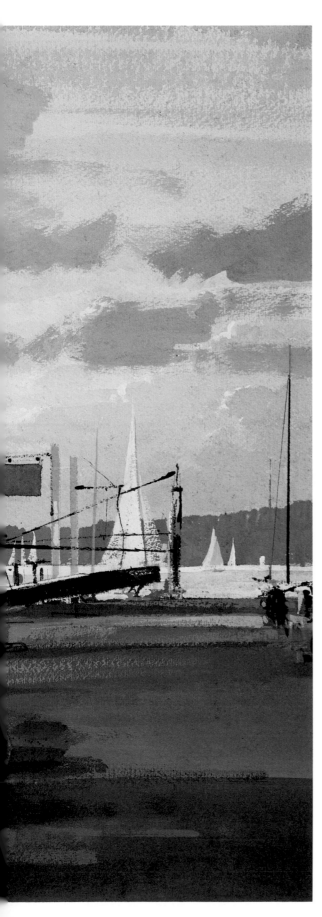

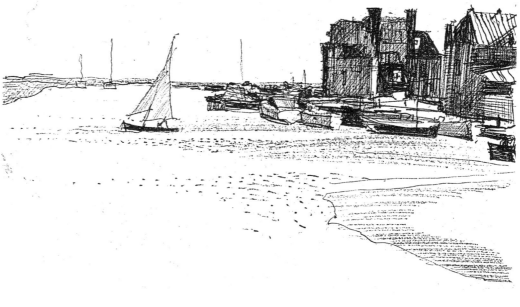

BIRDHAM POOL   (*Overleaf*) MINSMERE MARSHES, SUFFOLK

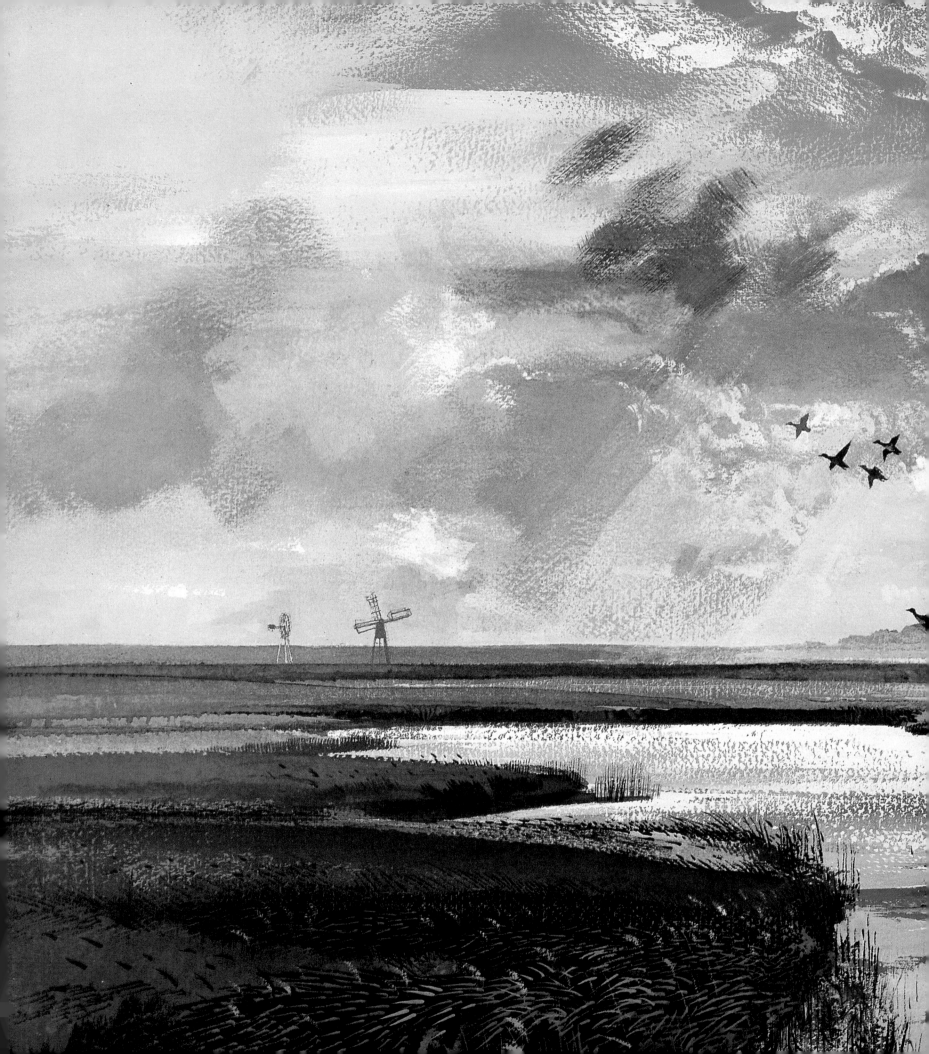

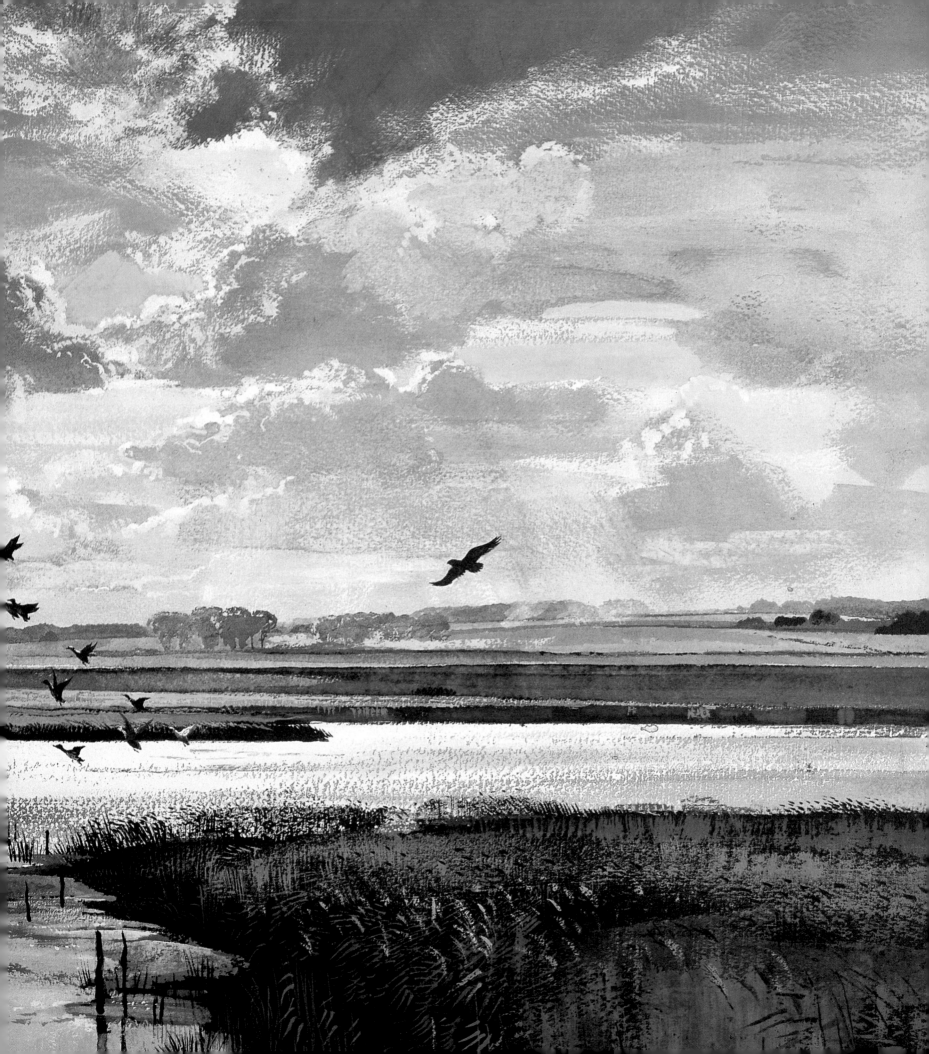

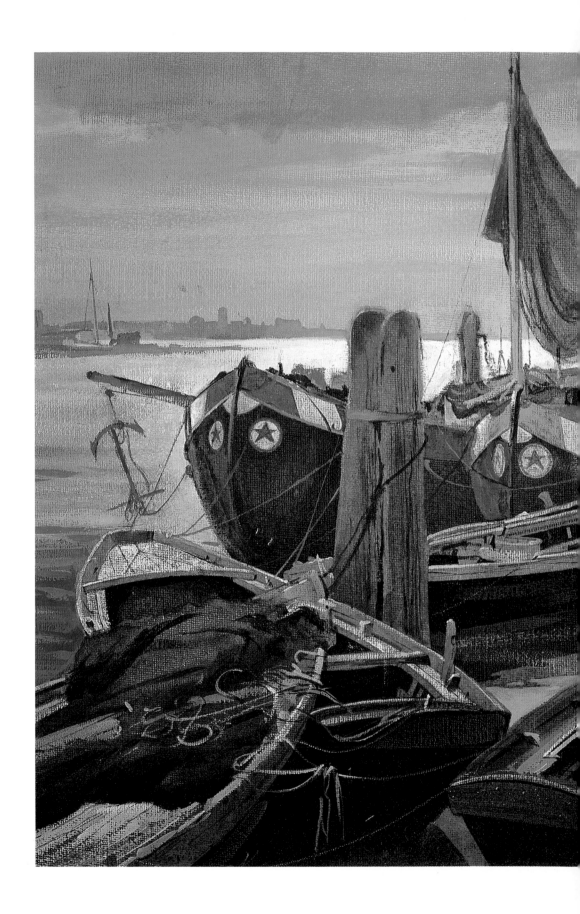

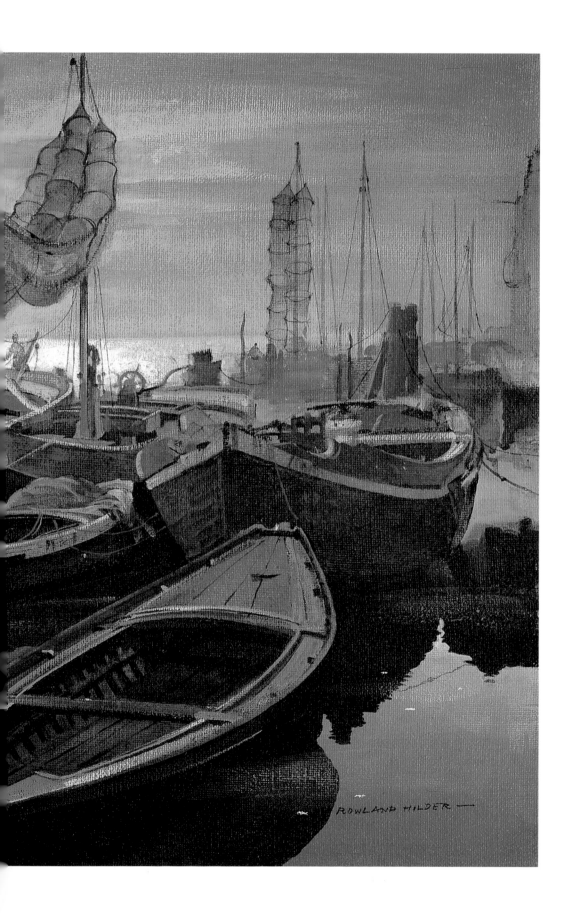

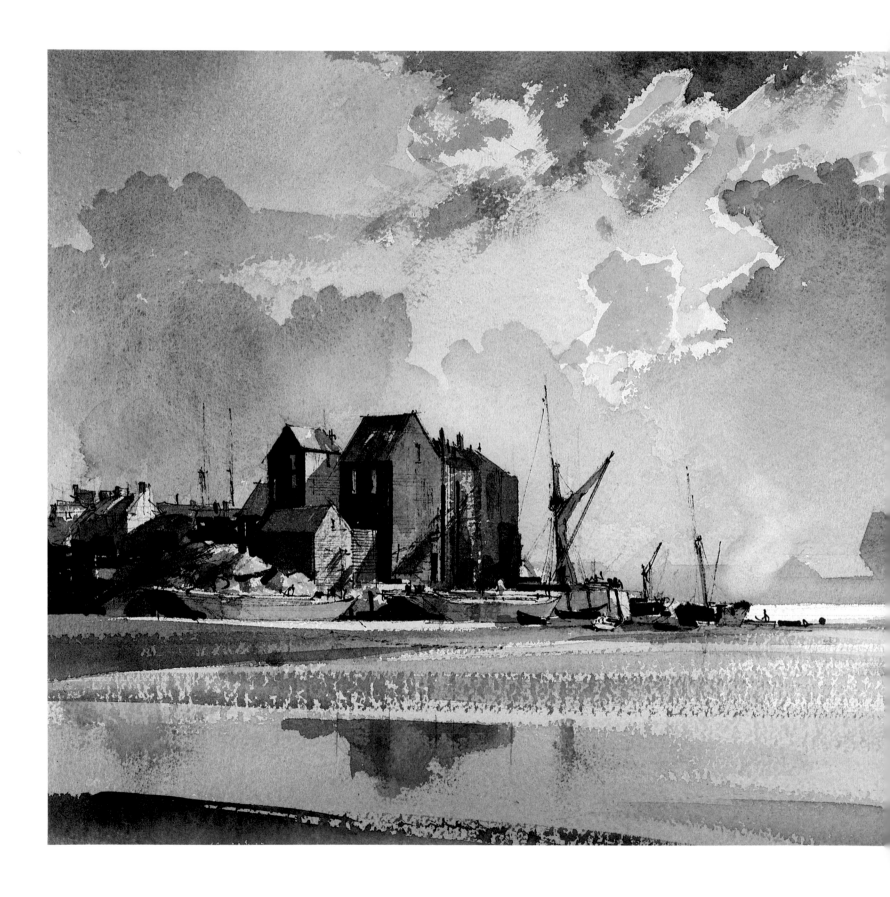

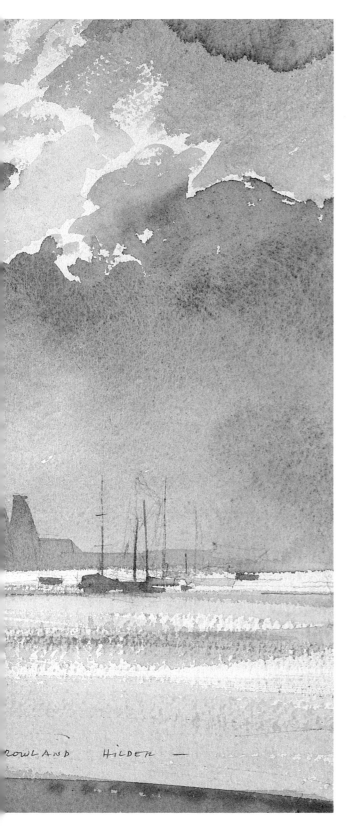

ROWLAND HILDER —

'One thing one learns as time passes is that dogmas and the received wisdom of teachers and art scholars are ephemeral.'

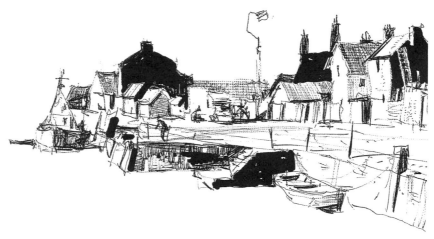

THE RIVER SWALE AT QUEENBOROUGH, KENT

The Medway is Kent's own river. By the time it merges with the estuary of the Thames it is wide and tidal, flowing through vast marshlands, loud with wildfowl. The town of Queenborough, named after Queen Eleanor of Castile, is still one of the remotest places in southern England. Its days were numbered when the sailing barges no longer brought business and cargoes to its very doors. The Swale remains, as a sea river, a challenging waterway for yachtsmen, and it is the Swale that makes an island of Sheppey.

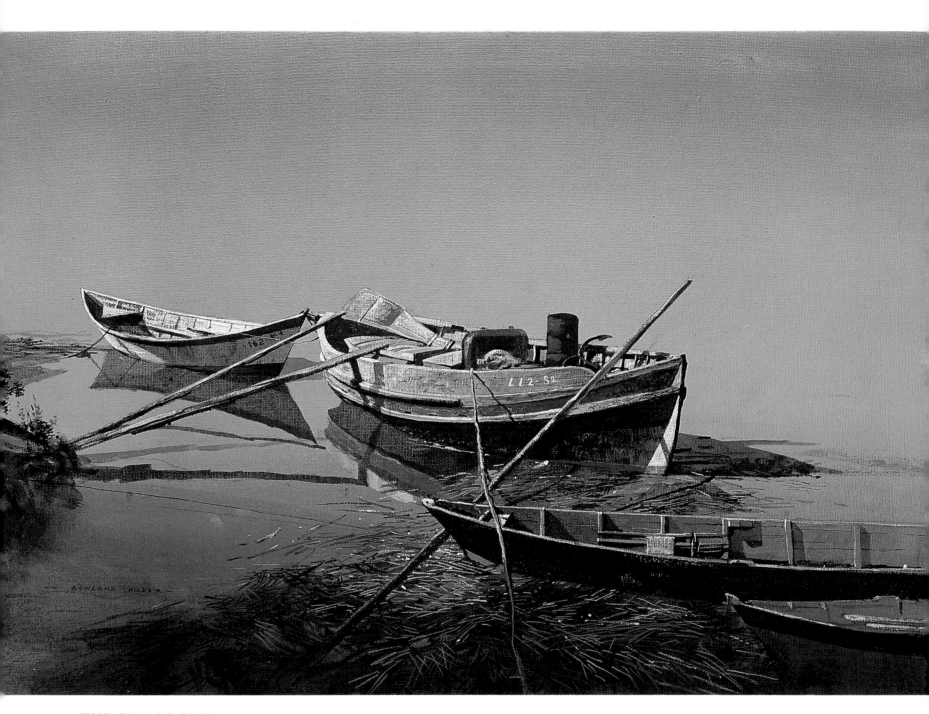

THE CAMARGUE

PEN AND PENCIL

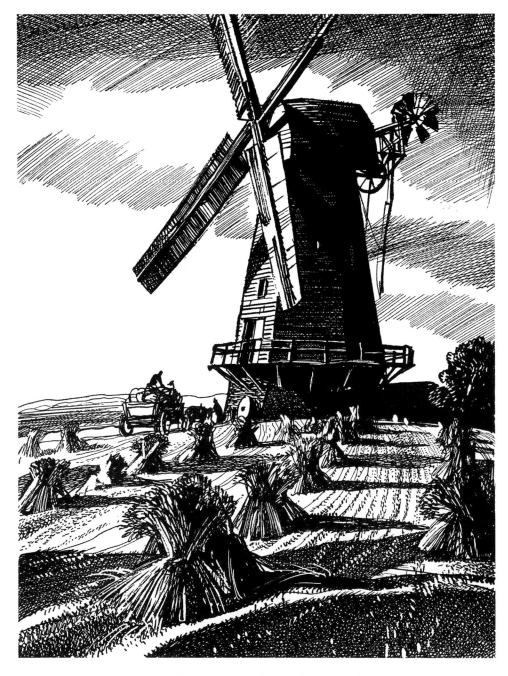

'Giving to the Common Land Fruitfulness and Beauty.'
From *The Bible for Today*, 1942.

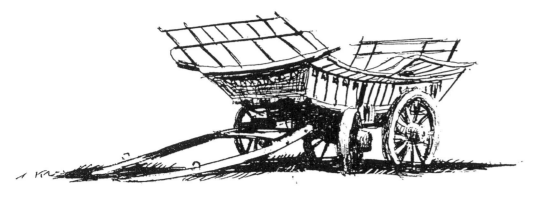

In the village of Birling, near Maidstone, Kent (*below right*), lived my grandmother, Ellen, in whose cottage next to the butcher's shop and the old Bull Inn (*right*) I spent the summers of my childhood. She was born in the cottage in Horn Street, of which I made this sketch (*below*) for a little book on Birling which was privately published in 1982 in aid of the church-tower fund.

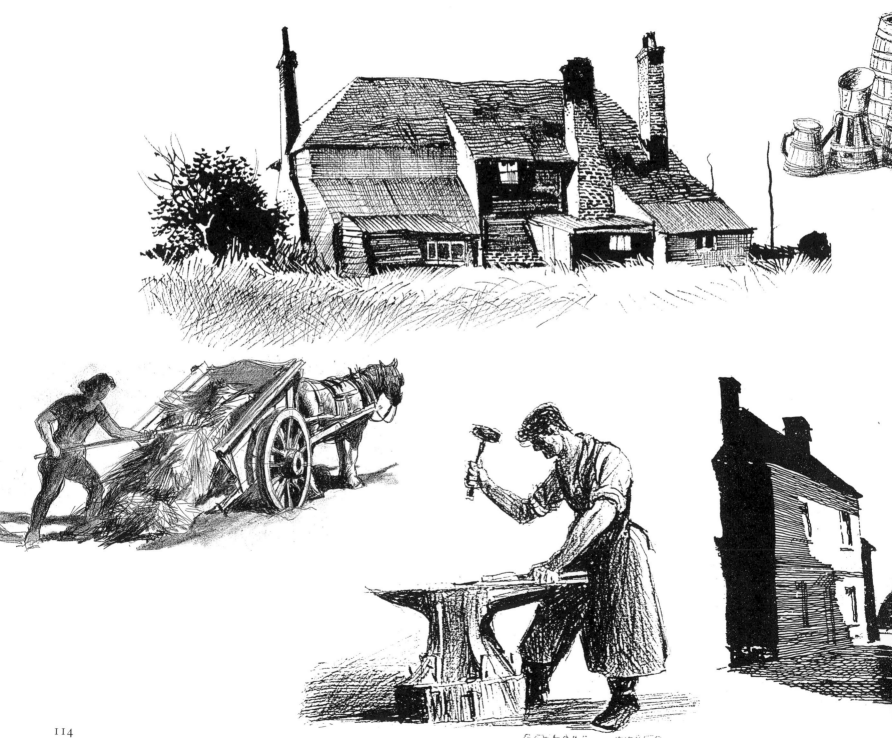

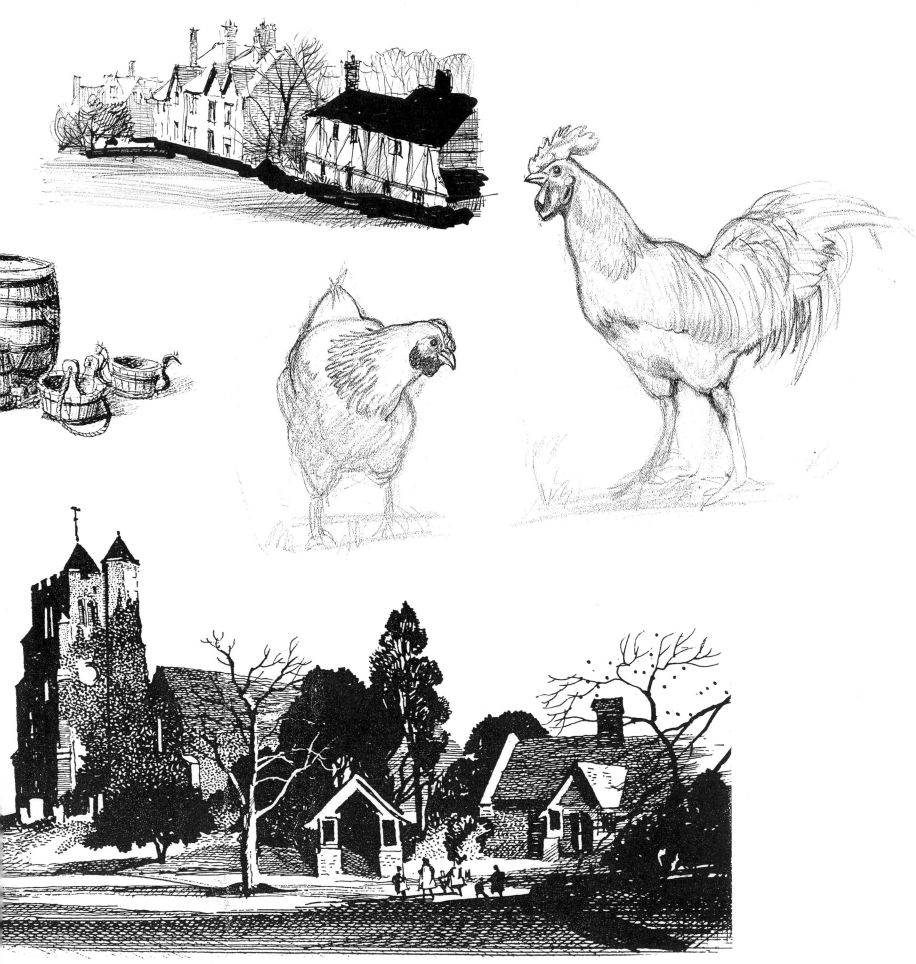

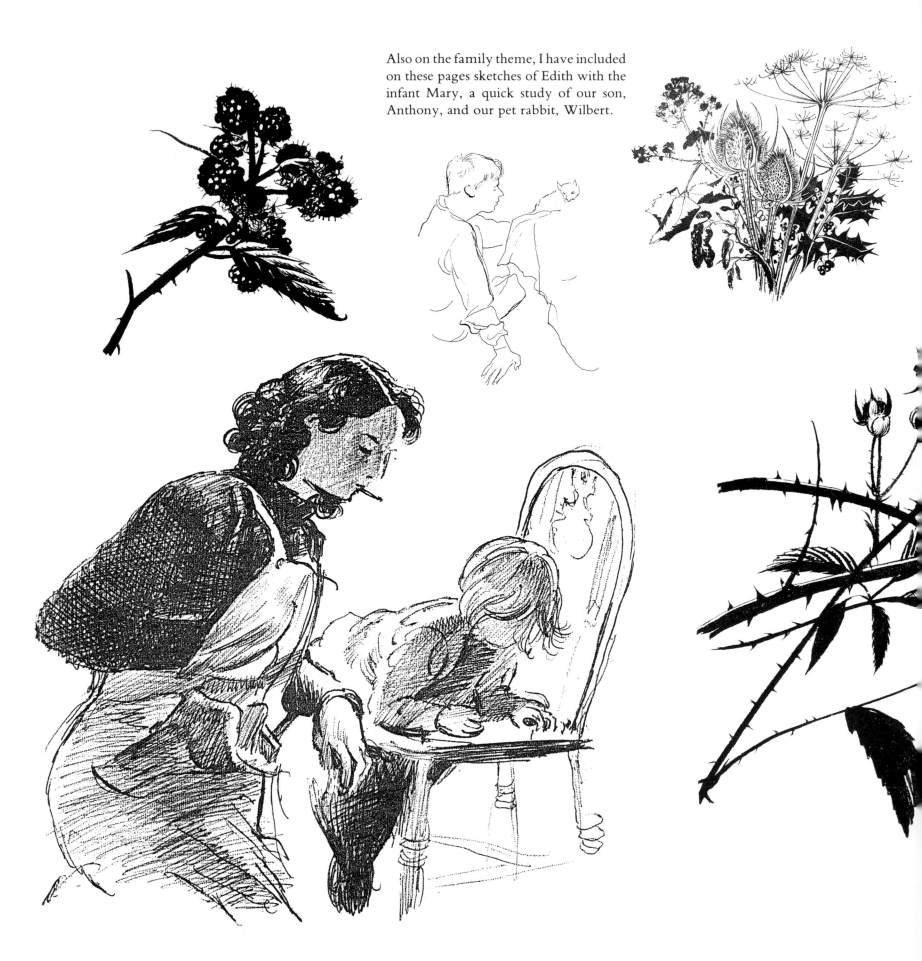

Also on the family theme, I have included on these pages sketches of Edith with the infant Mary, a quick study of our son, Anthony, and our pet rabbit, Wilbert.

The 'Flowers of the Countryside' series was to break new ground. Day after day, Edith and I would set off together, looking for specimens. We found them, usually in rainstorms or howling gales, refusing to keep still and be painted. Here are some of Edith's flower studies, and a 'rough' in which I sketched a possible landscape background for January. We then turned our respective contributions into finished artwork.

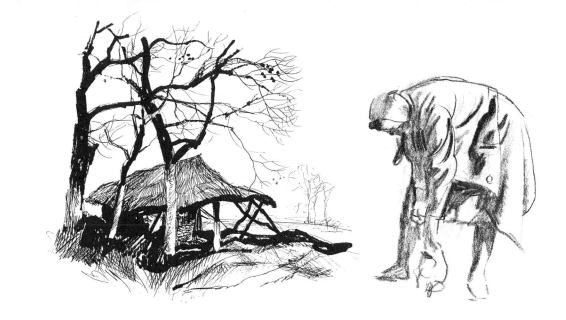

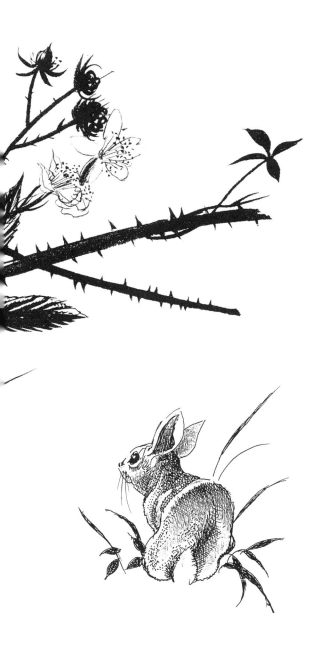

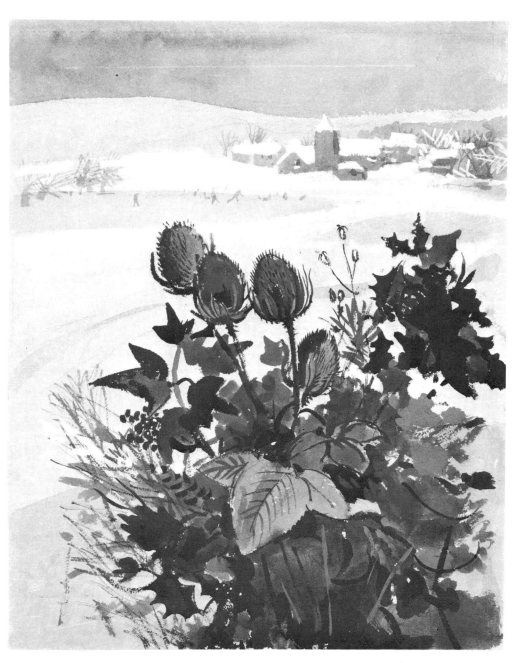

'I was taught to use a sketching pad as a reporter uses
his shorthand notebook, always at hand whatever the subject.
The essential thing was to catch the passing scene.'

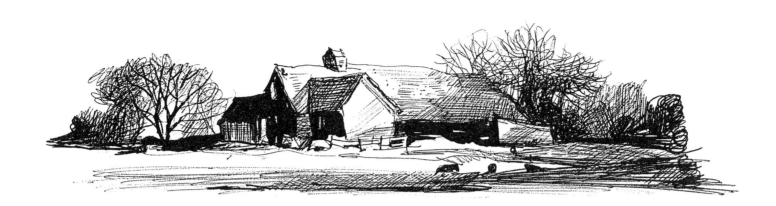

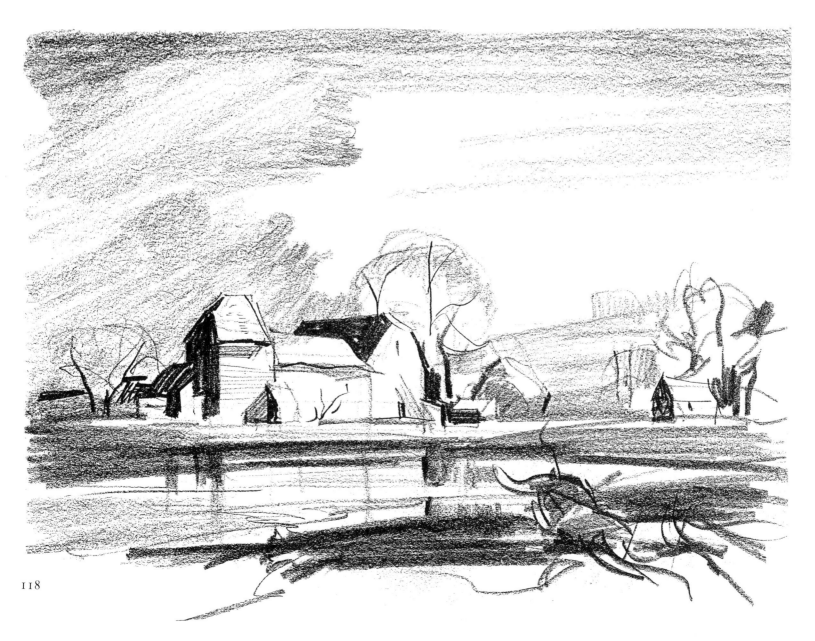

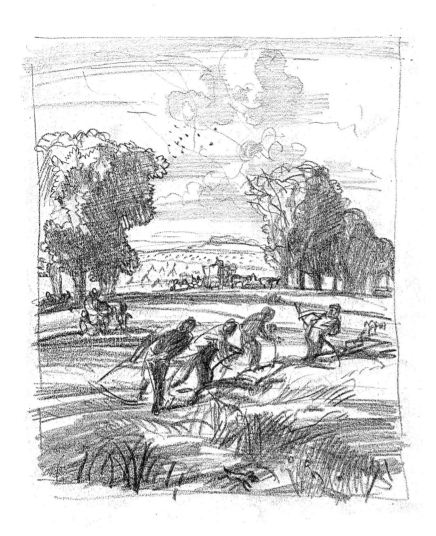
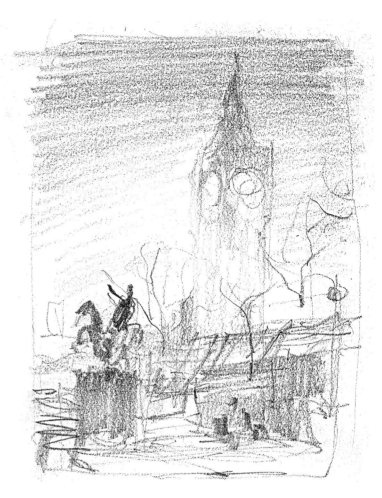
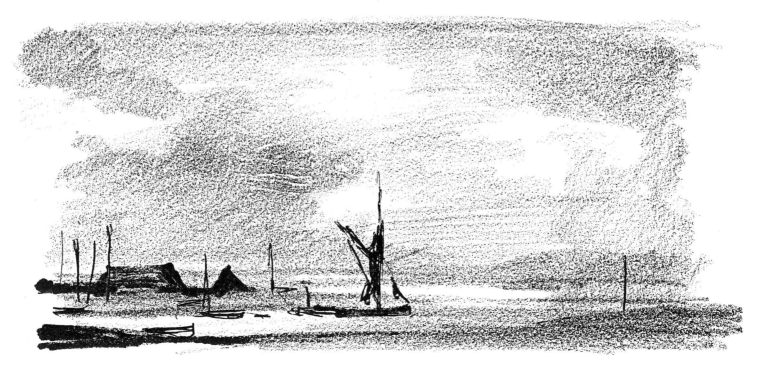

At art college I started in the etching class. That knowledge of the medium lay dormant until recent times, when it has provided me with an additional means of expression by enabling me to re-work some of my subjects as original limited-edition prints, from softground etchings to aquatints – and, most recently, introducing the now-respectable element of colour.

This version of *A Norfolk Farm*, shown as a watercolour on page 17, is an etching with aquatint, produced in a limited edition in 1985 with the help of my son-in-law, Rado Klose, who mans the proofing press in our basement at Blackheath.

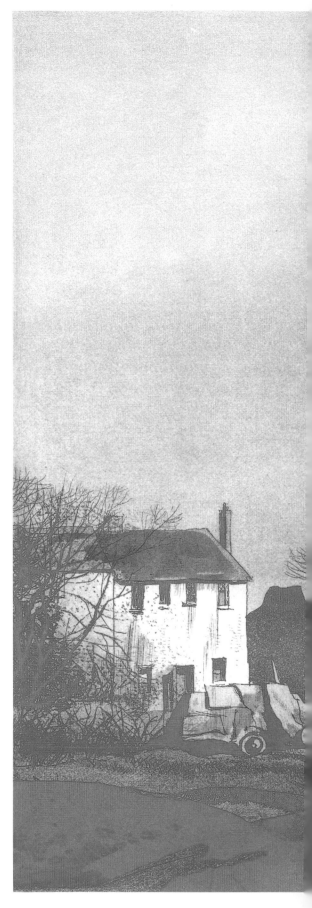

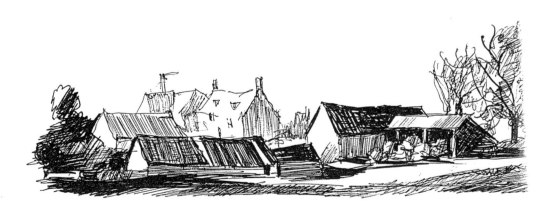

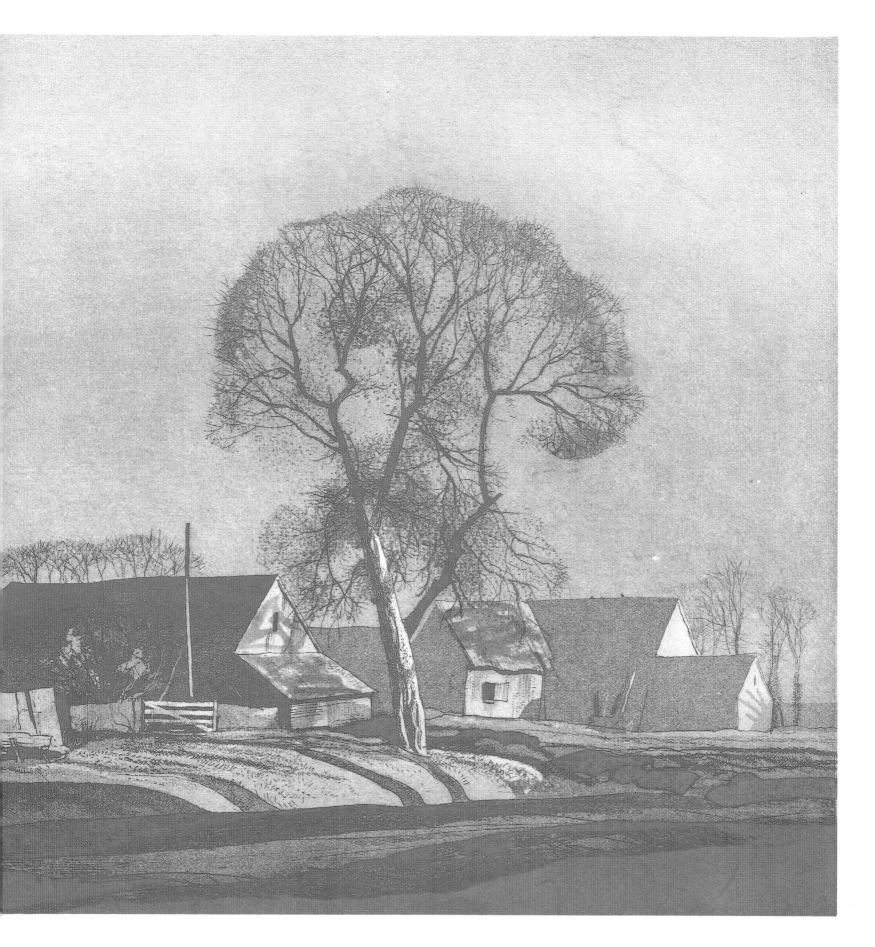

'The Shoreham Valley, which is at the heart of what people now call the Samuel Palmer country, is also at the heart of much of my work.'

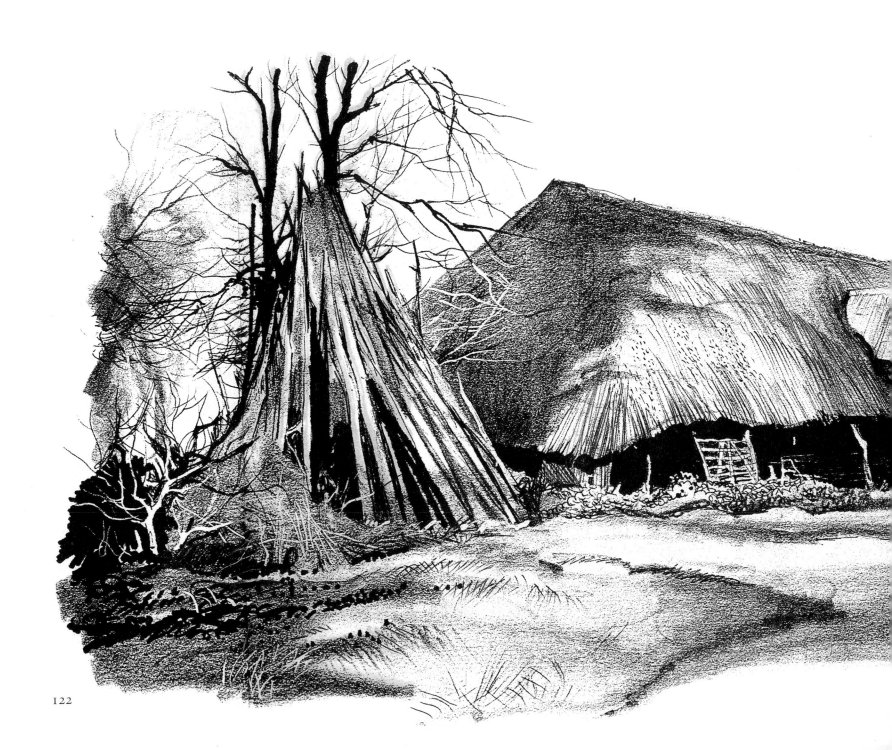

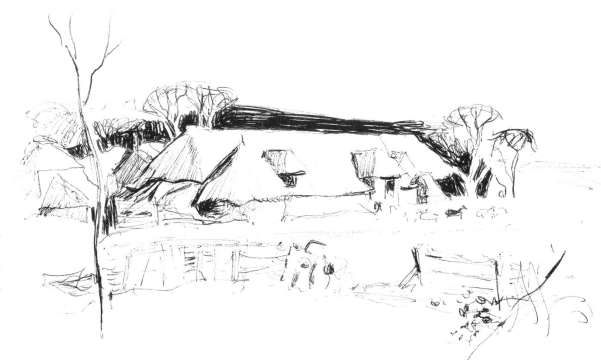

This drawing is a recollection of the old barn at Sepham Farm, in the Shoreham Valley, just as Samuel Palmer painted it in the 1820s and as I came across it a hundred years later, complete with hop-poles, old farm implements, and a haystack. Palmer's version, which I have roughly copied here for comparison, is now in the Paul Mellon collection.

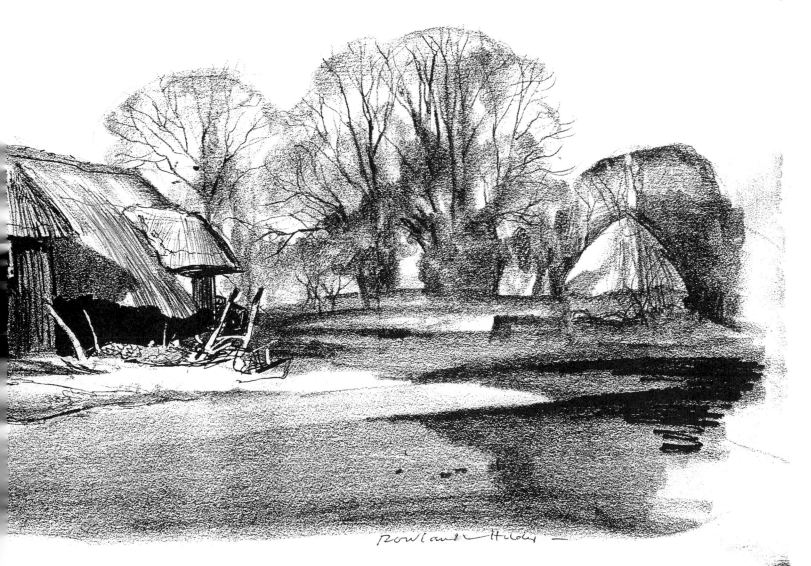

123

'The Thames was alive with activity,

men's shouts sounding above the cry of the gulls . . .'

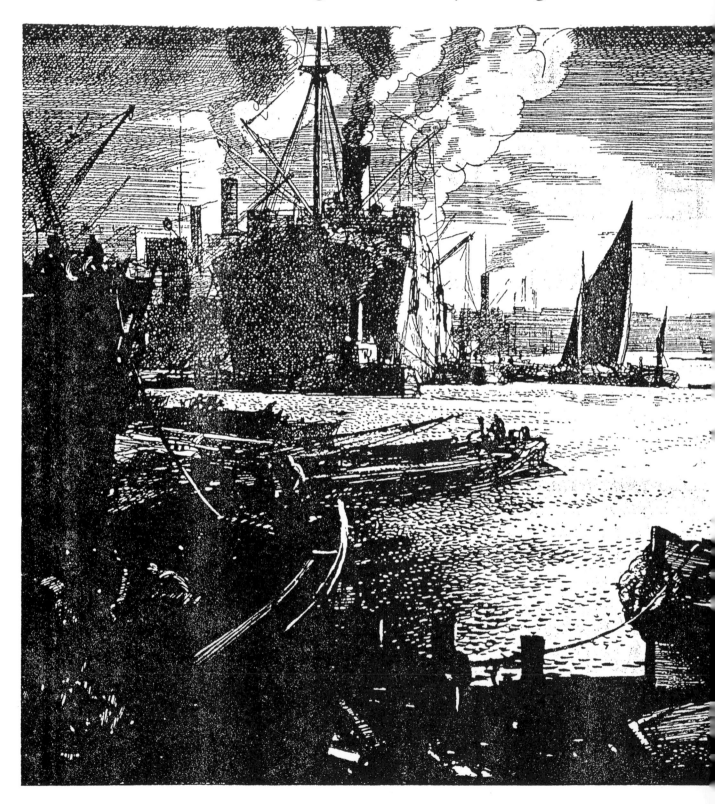

A double-spread of London Docks, drawn for *The Bible for Today*, 1942.

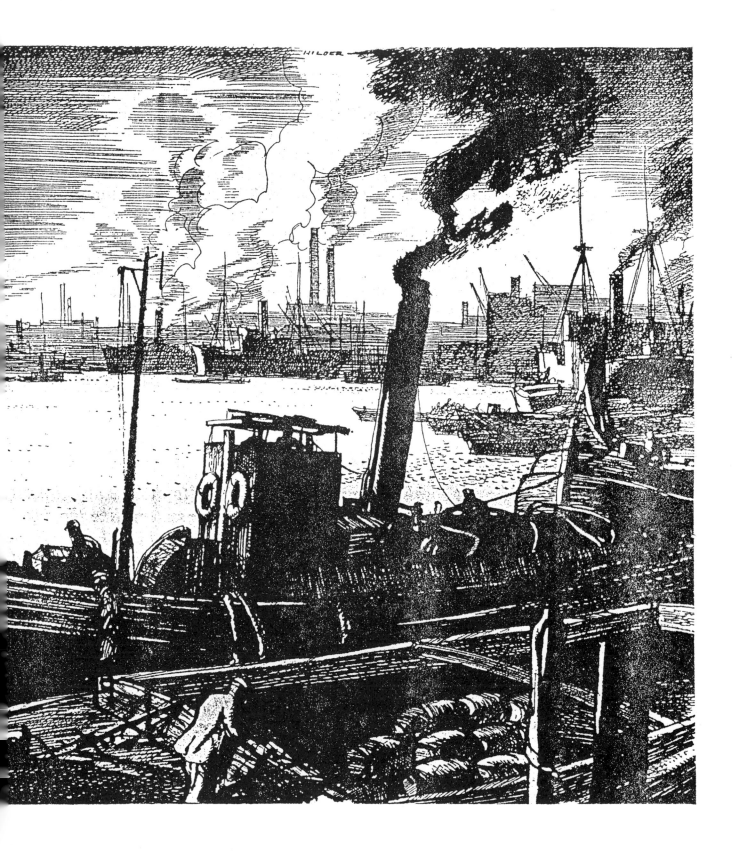

'Every repetition of what people call Hilderscapes
is really another variant on an inexhaustible theme.'

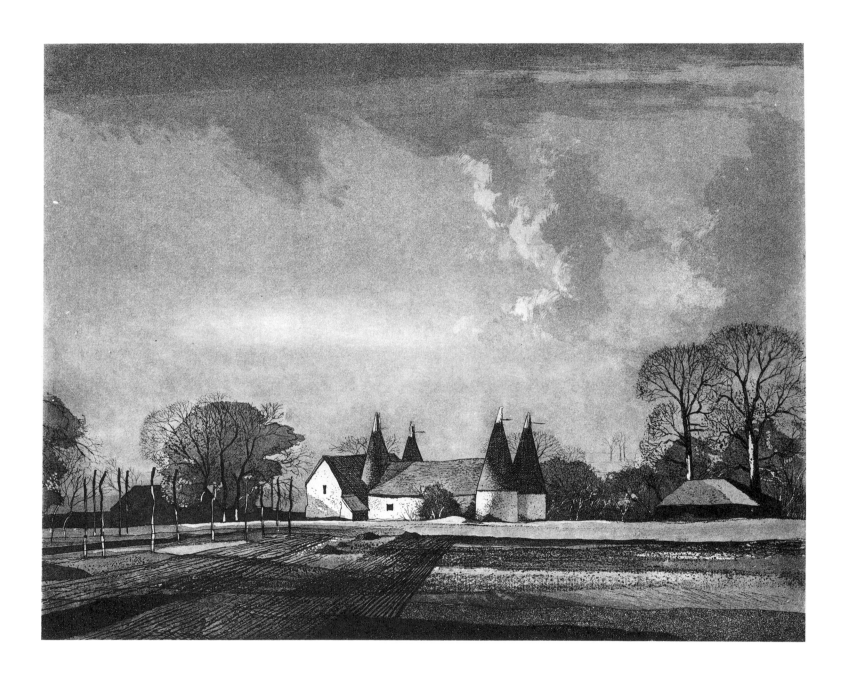

BIBLIOGRAPHY

BOOKS BY ROWLAND HILDER

Starting with Watercolour Studio Vista 1966

Painting Landscapes in Watercolour Collins 1983

Rowland Hilder's England The Herbert Press 1986

BOOKS ILLUSTRATED BY ROWLAND HILDER

The Riddle of the Air Percy F. Westerman, Blackie 1925

Moby Dick Herman Melville, Jonathan Cape 1926

The Adventures of a Trafalgar Lad John Lesterman, Jonathan Cape 1926

The Junior Cadet Percy F. Westerman, Blackie 1927

A Sailor of Napoleon John Lesterman, Jonathan Cape 1927

A Pair of Rovers John Lesterman, Jonathan Cape 1928

The Second Mate of the Myradale John Lesterman, Jonathan Cape 1929

Treasure Island Robert Louis Stevenson 1929

Then and Now Shell Mex Ltd 1929

Precious Bane Mary Webb, Jonathan Cape 1929

Kidnapped Robert Louis Stevenson, Oxford University Press 1930

The Senior Cadet Percy F. Westerman, Blackie 1931

Little Peter the Great H. A. Manhood, Jackson 1931

The Midnight Folk John Masefield, Heinemann 1931

Three Tales of the Sea C. Fox-Smith, Oxford University Press 1932

In Defence of British Rivers, Shell Mex and BP Ltd 1932

Fire Down Below W. M. W. Watt, Muller 1935

They Went to the Island L. A. G. Strong, Dent 1940

In collaboration: *The Bible for Today*, Oxford University Press 1941

In collaboration with Edith Hilder: *The Shell Guide to Flowers of the Countryside* Geoffrey Grigson, Phoenix House 1955

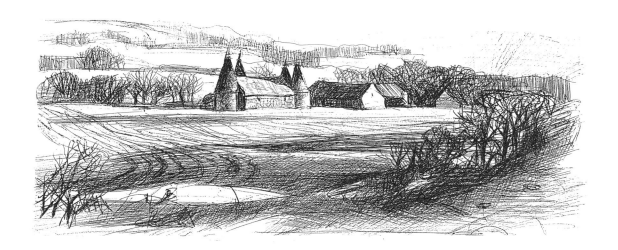

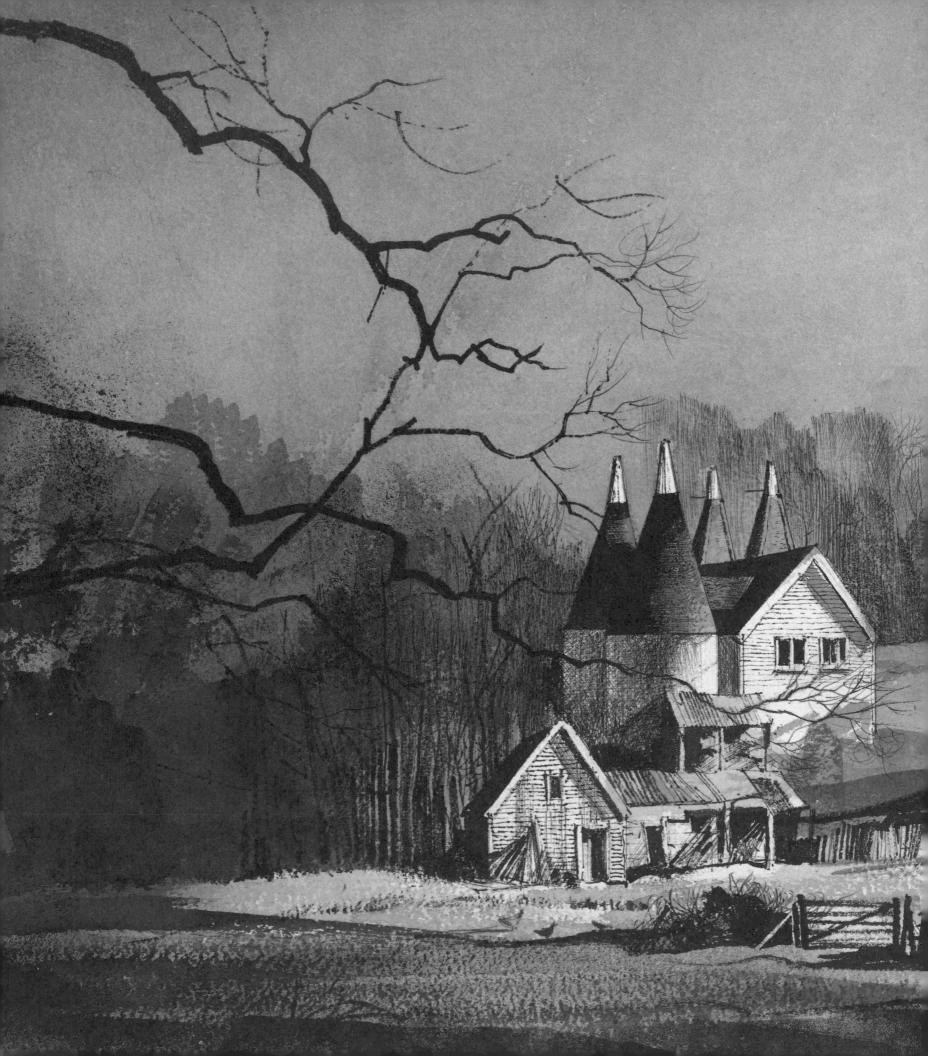